Tests and Measurements in Speech-Language Pathology

Tests and Measurements in Speech-Language Pathology

Edited by

Dennis M. Ruscello, Ph.D.

Professor of Speech-Language Pathology and Audiology, West Virginia University, Morgantown; Adjunct Professor of Otolaryngology, Robert C. Byrd Health Sciences Center, Morgantown

with 7 contributing authors

BUTTERWORTH
HEINEMANN

Boston Oxford Auckland Johannesburg Melbourne New Delhi

MW

AMERICAN FORESTS
GLOBAL
ReLEAF
2000

Butterworth–Heinemann supports the efforts of American Forests and the Global ReLeaf program in its campaign for the betterment of trees, forests, and our environment.

Library of Congress Cataloging-in-Publication Data
Tests and measurements in speech-language pathology / edited by Dennis M. Ruscello.
    p. ; cm.
  Includes index.
  ISBN 0-7506-7003-7
   1. Communicative disorders—Diagnosis. I. Ruscello, Dennis M.
   [DNLM: 1. Speech Disorders—diagnosis. 2. Language Disorders—diagnosis. 3.
Speech-Language Pathology. WV 500 T345 2000]
  RC423 .T435 2000
  6163.85'5075—dc21

                                                                00-046751

British Library Cataloguing-in-Publication Data
A catalogue record for this book is available from the British Library.

The publisher offers special discounts on bulk orders of this book.
For information, please contact:

Manager of Special Sales
Butterworth-Heinemann
225 Wildwood Avenue
Woburn, MA 01801-2041
Tel: 781-904-2500
Fax: 781-904-2620

For information on all Butterworth–Heinemann publications available,
contact our World Wide Web home page at: http://www.bh.com

10 9 8 7 6 5 4 3 2 1

Printed in the United States of America

7/19/02

This book is dedicated to my family:
Edie, Scott, Craig, and Mark

Contents

Contributing Authors

Mary Boyle, Ph.D., CCC-SLP, BC-NCD
Director of Speech-Language Pathology and Audiology, Burke Rehabilitation Hospital, White Plains, New York

Carl A. Coelho, Ph.D.
Associate Professor of Communication Sciences, University of Connecticut, Storrs

Thomas A. Crowe, Ph.D.
Professor and Chair of Communicative Disorders and Director of the Center for Speech and Hearing Research, The University of Mississippi, Oxford

Ronald B Gillam, Ph.D.
Associate Professor of Communication Sciences and Disorders, The University of Texas at Austin

LaVae M. Hoffman, Ph.D., CCC-SLP
Independent Consultant, Austin, Texas

Tommie L. Robinson, Jr., Ph.D.
Assistant Professor of Pediatrics, George Washington University School of Medicine and Health Sciences, Washington, DC; Director of Scottish Rite Center for Childhood Language Disorders, Hearing and Speech Center, Children's National Medical Center, Washington, DC

Dennis M. Ruscello, Ph.D.
Professor of Speech-Language Pathology and Audiology, West Virginia University, Morgantown; Adjunct Professor of Otolaryngology, Robert C. Byrd Health Sciences Center, Morgantown

A. Lynn Williams, Ph.D.
Associate Professor of Communicative Disorders, East Tennessee State University, Johnson City

Preface

The diagnosis of communication and related disorders is a major responsibility of the speech-language pathologist. The tools, which include various performance tests and measurements, are used in conjunction with other clinical data to develop an accurate assessment of a patient. This book provides a discussion of tests and measurements from the perspective of practitioners who have seen large numbers of clients and have also engaged in research with specific patient groups. It is the combination of professional practice and scholarship that makes each author special and his or her contribution unique to the speech-language pathology literature.

In the introductory chapter, I have articulated the position that diagnosis is an intellectual process of the highest degree, and one's diagnostic skills are constantly evolving. Practitioners use their problem-solving strategies to collect, analyze, and interpret the performance data collected from the patient and caregivers. The problem-solving strategies evolve over time, because the practitioner is constantly expanding his or her professional experience and engaging in life-long learning activities that enhance diagnostic skills. A framework for diagnosis includes the theoretical model of the disorder, because the model dictates the various tests and measurements that will be used. After data collection, the speech-language pathologist must interpret the data using professional judgment to arrive at a diagnosis. The position is made that tests and measurements are the primary data collection tools of the practitioner, but the professional judgment of the practitioner is the important component of the diagnostic process. The authors of the individual chapters discuss tests and measurements within a framework that allows the practitioner to identify the disorder and describe the major features of the disorder.

In Chapter 2, Williams discusses the assessment of phonological disorders. Sound system disorders constitute a major portion of the caseload of many practitioners. The author takes the position that the practitioner needs to discover the rules and patterns of a patient's phonological system. Although a patient may have a significant problem, specific rules and patterns are used and need to be identified. The use of specific assessment tools provides the raw data that will be used in the phonological analysis. Williams further indicates that the patient dictates the type of analysis conducted on the test data. That is, the practitioner must analyze the patient's test responses in relation to the phonological disorder presented by the patient. The author's cogent examples provide the reader with a detailed account of the various analysis procedures that may be used on test data.

Gillam and Hoffman provide a succinct description of child language disorders and guide the reader through a very specific and detailed assessment model in Chapter 3. They underscore the fact that a language disorder can impact on literacy development, particularly the acquisition of reading. Similar to the position presented by Williams, Gillam and Hoffman stress that tests, measurements, and observations are the interpretive structures of the assessment process. For example, observation of the patient in different communicative contexts helps the speech-language pathologist understand the impact of the disorder on the child's communicative interactions. According to the authors, the areas of assessment include the patient's psychological structures underlying language, knowledge of language structures and functions, and communication use in various social interactions. The assessment model is an excellent blueprint for understanding the patient and making recommendations for management.

Chapter 4 is a very detailed discussion of tests and measurements used in the assessment of patients with adult language disorders. Coelho and Boyle guide the reader through the different tests and measurements and clearly discuss the advantages of using the tests with specific patient groups. The purpose of assessment is to identify the communicative strengths and weaknesses of the client so that a plan of rehabilitation may be undertaken. Coelho and Boyle also delineate patient factors that the practitioner should be cognizant of when conducting an assessment, because their position is that test selection can only be done by considering the communication milieu of the patient. Finally, Coelho and Boyle argue that treatment planning is a very complex process that emanates from thorough assessment.

Chapter 5 is devoted to assessment tests and measurements that are used with the speech disorders of fluency and voice. Robinson and Crowe review these instruments for the reader in a very cogent fashion. The authors are careful to remind that assessment must take multicultural influences into account, because there are differences among cultures that can influence the assessment. Their discussion of assessment tools affords a practitioner the opportunity to select commercial assessment materials that can be used with their patients, regardless of age. Assessments of fluency and voice are very challenging tasks, but Robinson and Crowe explain the positive and negative features of each test along with the implication of usage for each.

Chapter 6 deals exclusively with the oral-motor examination, a component of almost all communication and related assessments. I explain that inspection of the oral anatomy and physiology must be carried out in a systematic manner with careful attention to infection control. Identified variations in anatomy and physiology are not always causal factors in the development and maintenance of a speech disorder; however, such variations need to be identified. Chapter 6 includes a discussion of each articulator and potential problem that might be present in the population of patients seen by the speech-language pathologist. Although many practitioners carry out the assessment with their own materials, there are commercial tests that are available. These commercial tests are also reviewed in the chapter, and supplementary appendices that can be used for assessment are included for perusal.

Each chapter deals with a different communication disorder, but the common unifying factor is that each author independently states that tests and measurements provide a base for diagnosis. It is the interpretation of the data that is so important to the assessment. This book presents assessment as an intellectual endeavor and challenges the reader to use such a mind set in professional practice. Diagnosis is a constantly evolving process and a major responsibility of the practitioner.

D.M.R.

Tests and Measurements in Speech-Language Pathology

1 Use of Tests and Measurements in Speech-Language Pathology: An Introduction to Diagnosis

Dennis M. Ruscello

Diagnosis of communication and related disorders is a challenging process that is an integral part of practice. It is not simply the administration of various tests, measurements, and collection of observational data, but an intellectual process that includes the collection, integration, and interpretation of client data. The guiding force in the process is the professional judgment of the practitioner. The rationale for a diagnosis may differ as a function of the diagnostic question being asked. Depending on the client and the reason for assessment, the clinician may need to identify the presence of a communication disorder, specify the particular disorder type, or provide a prognosis for treatment. In many cases, the clinician must consider all of the questions when forming a diagnosis, because each of the diagnostic questions leads into the other. That is, the clinician first determines if there is a communication disorder. The existence of a disorder would then lead to the specification of the disorder type, and finally, the clinician would provide a recommendation for treatment of the disorder.

Campbell (1998) described the diagnostic process as one of the most complex and difficult responsibilities for the practitioner. He suggested that clinicians use different problem-solving strategies to formulate an appropriate diagnosis. That is, the use of professional judgment in diagnosis may reflect different strategies on the part of the practitioner.

Sackett et al. (1991) have identified four basic strategies that are typically used by clinicians to render clinical diagnoses. The first strategy is known as *pattern recognition*. A patient presents with certain characteristics, which are indicative of a particular pattern associated with a communication disorder. For example, a child with spastic cerebral palsy would suggest the presence of a dysarthria. Confirmation of the disorder and identification of the major characteristics would then need to be delineated through an assessment of the patient's speech characteristics. Practitioners who have extensive clinical experience often use a pattern recognition strategy when engaging in diagnosis because of their familiarity with a variety of clinical cases.

A second strategy, multiple-branching or arborization, is another strategy that is used by some practitioners. A diagnosis is made by considering symptoms in the context of a decision-making tree or matrix. The clinician follows an algorithm to arrive at the appropriate diagnosis. Campbell (1998) indicated that practitioners without extensive experience might use such a strategy, because all possible alternatives are included for scrutiny. Yoder and Kent (1988) compiled a set of arborization strategies, which may be used in the diagnosis of communication and other related disorders. Practitioners with expertise in particular areas developed algorithms that can be used by clinicians for diagnosis. A practitioner would follow the algorithm by obtaining certain diagnostic information and using those data to make diagnostic decisions.

A third diagnostic strategy is diagnosis by exhaustion. As implied, the client undergoes a battery of tests and measurements and is subject to the collection of an extensive case history. This strategy can be quite time-consuming, because the practitioner is attempting to establish a diagnosis by eliminating all possible alternatives. Novice clinicians may find this strategy appealing, because it furnishes an inclusive approach to eliminating potential diagnoses and identifying the accurate one. However, such an approach can be very inefficient in terms of cost and client testing.

The fourth and final strategy is the hypothetico-deductive approach. The practitioner uses a deductive reasoning approach to eliminate diagnoses that may share certain characteristics with the correct diagnosis. Diagnostic procedures are modified during the evaluation as the clinician arrives at the correct diagnosis. Experienced clinicians who are well versed in understanding the various disorders and symptoms of the disorders generally use this approach to diagnosis because of their extensive background and knowledge of speech and language disorders.

Although not presented in a hierarchy, the problem-solving strategies reflect to some extent levels of experience and expertise with certain diagnostic entities. Practitioners may use different strategies that vary as a function of the client and their own level of professional expertise. A particular client may present with a constellation of problems that are quite familiar to the practitioner; consequently, a diagnostic strategy of pattern recognition might be used. Conversely, a client with a pattern of problems not seen on a frequent basis may require a multiple-branching strategy, so that alternative diagnoses may be eliminated in favor of the appropriate diagnosis.

Regardless of the diagnostic strategy, the clinician uses various tests and measurements to estimate the client's performance level on various speech, language, and related instruments (Hegde, 1996). Other relevant information, such as case history data, needs to be collected so that an appropriate diagnosis may be made. However, it is to be stressed that the actual diagnosis is a function of the practitioner's clinical skills. Decisions are made on the basis of data interpretation, not simply the collection of data. It is the professional judgment of the practitioner that is used to form the diagnosis and communicate the findings to the patient and care-givers through verbal discussion and written report.

This book presents reference tests and measurements that are representative of those used in speech-language pathology. There have been such publications in the past, but they have generally been categorizations of assessment instruments without an underlying plan for actual assessment and subsequent diagnosis. The authors of the different chapters are expert in specific areas of speech-language pathology, and each presents an underlying theoretical model for the assessment of the different disorders, along with a diagnostic process. It is within this theory/process rationale that the diagnosis evolves as it guides the clinician in the collection of case history information and the selection and interpretation of tests and measurements. The accurate diagnosis of clients with communication or related disorders is an intellectual process of the highest degree. It is one of the cornerstones of professional practice and fosters the development of a plan for treatment.

Deputy and Weston (1998) developed a good example of a diagnostic framework in their conceptualization of the differential diagnosis of phonological disorders. The underlying or guiding theory was the one developed by Shriberg and Kwiatkowski (1982), who characterized the diagnosis of a phonological disorder as a comprehensive description of a client's speech involvement in relation to a number of additional speech and non-speech variables. Deputy and Weston used the theory to develop a diagnostic plan that could be used by practitioners. The assessment process involved the collection of client data that included both speech production and potential causal correlate information. Various tests, measurements, and other diagnostic information that could be used to make a differential diagnosis were discussed. Sample data were then carefully scrutinized to arrive at an appropriate diagnosis. This chapter deals with basic introductory issues of evaluation that are important in the conduct of a diagnostic assessment.

Diagnosis of Communication and Related Disorders

Meitus (1983) wrote that diagnosis is a clinical decision made by the practitioner in response to a problem or problems displayed by a particular client. A diagnosis is formulated through very careful scrutiny of case history, examination, and observational data. Peterson and Marquardt (1990) characterized diagnosis as a descriptive task that the practitioner must carry out in everyday practice. The features of the disorder are specified through evaluation, so that the clinician may determine the overall communication and related abilities and disabilities of the client. Presenting conditions or factors that are found to coexist must also be identified because they may affect the disorder. For example, a client may have undergone a diagnostic evaluation, and the results of testing indicated hyponasal speech. The feature of the disorder was identified through the evaluation; however, the clinician also needs to identify any factors that may contribute to the problem. Habitual mouth breathing noted in the case history and observations of an open mouth posture during the diagnostic evaluation indicate a med-

TABLE 1.1   A model for the diagnosis of communication and related disorders

Theoretical model used to conceptualize the disorder
Process variables
   Case history information
   Tests and measurements
Interpretation of diagnostic information
Professional judgment

ical referral to examine the nose, nasopharynx, and midface for some type of nasal obstruction or midface growth deficiency. Confirmation of such a problem would lead the clinician to conclude that medical intervention may be necessary to eliminate the hyponasality.

The subsequent sections of this chapter present an overview of variables that constitute the diagnostic process. Table 1.1 summarizes a proposed framework for diagnosis and includes the theoretical model used in conceptualizing the disorder, the process variables or information to be collected, and the outcome or interpretation of the collected data. An additional variable that needs to be considered is the clinical or professional judgment of the clinician in solving the diagnostic problem. Although it is an abstract construct and problematic to objectify, professional judgment is the important component of the diagnostic process (Sackett et al., 1991). The clinician must use professional judgment if an accurate diagnosis is to be made. The remaining portion of this chapter discusses case history information, tests and measurements, interpretation of diagnostic information, and professional judgment issues.

Historical data can be collected from the patient and caregiver. This furnishes information that helps the practitioner diagnose the disorder. The actual performance of the client is evaluated through the use of various tests and measurements. There are many different types of tests, observational scales, and other tools that may be used in the diagnostic assessment. The selection of such tests and measurements depends on the client and the theoretical model underlying the practitioner's conceptualization of the particular disorder. After all diagnostic information has been collected, the practitioner must evaluate the resultant data and provide a diagnosis. The diagnosis is a professional judgment that is based on the client's performance and the clinical experience of the practitioner. Diagnosis is a process that is a composite of many factors. The process is continually evolving as the practitioner gains experience and the profession is constantly adding to its body of knowledge.

Process Variable: Case History

The case history is a body of information that is obtained to help the clinician understand the client and the client's communication and/or related disorder. Hegde (1996) indicated that the case history is a detailed account

TABLE 1.2   A summary of information typically collected through case history interview

Complaint
Referral source
History of the problem
    Factors associated with onset
    Factors associated with development and maintenance
    Previous diagnostic findings
    Treatment history
General developmental status and milestones
Current health
Educational/vocational status
Emotional/social status
Family dynamics
Other relevant information

that varies depending on the age of the client and the disorder. Areas of data gathering may include information pertaining to the client, such as occupation, disorder, development and health, education, family, and any additional information that is deemed appropriate. Generally, history information is collected through a standardized written form, personal interview, or both. It should be noted that there are many variations that are used in clinical practice. Some clinicians have the client or caregiver complete a standardized written case history before the actual evaluation. The information is then forwarded to the clinician for perusal. In some cases, a phone contact follows to seek clarity on certain queries and obtain additional information. In other cases, the preassessment information forms the basis for conducting a personal interview. Obtaining the history information before the evaluation enables the practitioner to plan the diagnostic testing and assign other professionals to the client, if necessary.

Complaint and Referral Source

Table 1.2 is an outline of data that are typically collected in a case history. The first bit of information is the complaint, or the reason for seeking the diagnostic evaluation. The complaint is the client's description of the problem. If the client is unable to describe the problem because of the communication disorder or because of his or her age, the caregiver needs to furnish the information. In either case, it is important to record the exact words of the client or caregiver. An adult client with a swallowing disorder might state that a diagnostic evaluation was requested because he or she "chokes when eating hard crunchy foods." A caregiver might indicate that his or her child is difficult to understand, and there is concern because the child will begin kindergarten shortly. The referral source also needs to be specified for the history. A physician, health care agency, colleague, or caregiver may have initiated the request for a diagnostic evaluation, and the results and recommendations of the evaluation need to be sent to the referral source.

Onset, Development, and Maintenance

The history of the problem provides a basis for understanding the impact of the disorder on the client and can also provide information that may be associated with the cause of the problem. Although it is often difficult to establish a causal relationship between a communication disorder and some co-occurring condition, history information related to the onset of the problem can be most valuable to the examiner. The client or caregiver should be questioned in regard to conditions that may be associated with the onset of the disorder. What factor or factors may be identified at onset? For example, a voice disorder may have occurred during a period of time in which the client engaged in abusive vocal behaviors, or in which an adult had a stroke with resultant aphasia. In other cases, establishing an association may not be possible because no specific factors can be associated with onset. For example, there may be no specific onset factors that can be associated with some children who exhibit language delay. Schery and Garber (1998) discuss the issues of differential diagnosis with this population and suggest that onset factors are not always forthcoming in the client history.

In addition to the onset of the disorder, information concerning development and maintenance needs to be gathered. That is, there needs to be a dialogue to explore the progress of the disorder since it was identified. Have the symptoms remained static, or have they increased in their severity? Are there periods of remission when the client is free from any symptoms, or are the variations marked by alterations in severity? These are questions that need to be asked when tracing the progression of a disorder. Moreover, the clinician needs to explore any factors that have been noted that may explain differences or variations in the disorder. There are numerous factors—such as medication changes, health status, environmental modifications, communication treatment, and other variables—that can cause changes in the communication disorder. It is only through careful history investigation that one can describe the progress of the disorder and isolate those reported factors judged responsible for any changes in the disorder.

Previous Diagnostic and Treatment Findings

Many patients who have been referred for a diagnostic evaluation have undergone other assessment(s). The previous results are germane to the current appraisal. What were the findings of the previous diagnostic evaluation(s)? Actual reports usually provide more reliable information and should be obtained rather than relying on the recollections of the client. In some cases, clients can accurately recall results, but in many cases, the information conveyed to the examiner is not accurate. Some clients hand carry clinical records for review by the examiner. Sometimes the examiner must request such records from other agencies, provided that appropriate client permission has been obtained. The perusal of such data enables the clinician to determine what was done and what recommendations were made. In addition, the clinician can determine if there is agreement or disparity with the past and current diagnostic findings. Meitus (1983) indicated that one should obtain all necessary diagnostic records. He further suggested that previous records were particularly important in the case of clients who showed extensive diagnostic histories with congruence among reported findings and recommendations. The repeated seeking of diagnostic services in light of similar findings and recommendations may signal the need for professional counseling.

If the client has received previous treatment services, the clinician should make note of such information. What was the result of the treatment that was conducted? The examiner can record verbal recollections; however, written summaries provide a more objective record of what was done therapeutically with the client and the client's response to the treatment. As discussed in regard to diagnostic findings, written report summaries enable the clinician to review the treatment methods, procedures, and results of previous therapy. The clinician can determine what was successful and what was not. Moreover, written reports can also assist the clinician in guiding the client or caregiver to the appropriate treatment services. Suffice to say that knowledge of previous services and the results of those services can be important diagnostic markers in some cases. Schery (1985) found that children with language disorders who had repeated clinical assessments without a diagnosis had a poorer prognosis for recovery than children with language disorders who had not undergone numerous diagnostic evaluations.

General Developmental Status

Information pertaining to the developmental status of the client varies as a function of age. When working with children and adolescents, it is often necessary to obtain a developmental history so that the examiner may study the communication disorder in relation to other developmental phenomena. Practitioners need to remember that speech and language develop in parallel to other developmental domains, such as cognition, fine and gross motor skills, and socioemotional adjustment (Owens, 1984). Moreover, development is a predictable process, with children achieving certain skills or abilities at predictable times. Although there is a substantial amount of variation among children, milestones are achieved as the child matures and is provided opportunities to learn. It is recommended that clinicians review developmental information and formulate questions that address specific aspects of development. Readers are referred to a number of excellent summaries that may be used for this purpose (Hegde, 1996; Kent, 1994; Owens, 1996). Generally, developmental data are not solicited from adult clients; rather, history is sought from the beginning of the reported symptoms to the present.

Cognition is one's intellect, and it allows a person to engage in a variety of mentalistic activities like communication (Owens, 1996). The developing child interacts with the environment to receive various types of input. Children perceive the incoming data differently, but they all categorize, store, and retrieve information to solve current and future problems. Moreover, their organization or way of dealing with environmental stimulation changes as a function of cognitive growth. The examiner should question the caregiver concerning milestone behaviors that reflect cognitive development. Some clients have undergone intellectual testing, and the results of the evaluation are available for the examiner. With other clients, the examiner may want to supplement historical information with a screening of nonverbal reasoning skills through the administration of a test or observational scale (Camarata & Swisher, 1990; Schery & Garber, 1998).

Another aspect of development is that of fine and gross motor skills (Rogers & Campbell, 1993). As neurologic and physical growth advance, the fine and gross motor skills of the child develop. He or she becomes involved with the environment and gradually develops control of small muscle groups (fine motor skills) and large muscle groups (gross motor skills). Some examples of fine motor control include coordinated skills associated with the eyes, hands, and fingers. Owens (1996) has indicated that fine motor skills gradually emerge and are generally refined by the early school years; however, some fine motor skills, such as mastery of finger control, are not attained until adulthood. Gross motor skills include the development of large muscles for activities such as walking, throwing, and running. The progression of gross motor skills is sequential, with little variability among children. The clinician can collect historical information and make observations concerning motor skills, but it may be necessary to request assessment from other professionals, such as occupational and physical therapists, when motor skills are in question.

A third developmental variable is socioemotional adjustment, or the growth and development of one's interactive skills with others. As the child grows and expands his or her realm of experience, there is a change from a generally egocentric individual to a more social individual who must interact with others in a variety of situations. The child gradually develops social behaviors that are guided by the social rules and customs of a particular society (Owens, 1996). It is important to remember the social aspect of communication and the potential effect of socioemotional maladjustment on communication. The examiner must explore this area with the caregiver to determine if there are any problems indicative of a socioemotional problem. Examiners may study socioemotional variables from intrapersonal and interpersonal perspectives. Intrapersonal adjustment consists of the client's feelings and attitudes about the communication disorder and other factors, such as the client's self-esteem and overall psychological state. Interpersonal factors pertain to the interactions of the client with others. That is, how does the client relate to others in the environment? As with other factors of the case history, this may be an area of important investigative study and potential referral (Stemple, 1998), or it may not warrant critical attention. The examiner must investigate thoroughly to determine if there is a relationship between the communication problem and the various developmental variables.

Current Health

Accurate information concerning the health of the patient is very important in providing a diagnosis, because there may be presenting conditions that alter how the diagnostic evaluation is carried out, indicate referrals to other specialties, or limit the prognosis for rehabilitation of the communicative disorder (Meitus, 1983). In some cases, testing conditions must be modified because of a specific problem that a patient might exhibit. For example, children referred for speech and language evaluations may also exhibit behavioral characteristics that are suggestive of attention-deficit/hyperactivity disorder (Bonem, 1994; Shaywitz et al., 1994; Weaver, 1993). The examiner needs to be aware of the condition and those behaviors that may interfere with the assessment process. Another example is the case in which there may be presenting conditions that require referral to other specialties, even if the speech-language pathologist diagnoses a communication disorder. For example, a client might present with a voice disorder and chronic cough requiring a referral for a medical examination and possible treatment. Finally, a significant medical condition may indicate a poor prognosis for the client, and this information must be factored into the findings and subsequent recommendations. For instance, a client who has a progressive neurologic disease, such as amyotrophic lateral sclerosis, would not have a positive prognosis for recovery of communicative functions, but recommendations could be made to maximize residual communication skills.

Educational/Vocational Status

The importance of the client's educational history depends on the communication disorder presented (Peterson & Marquardt, 1990). In some instances, it is not an important factor in the assessment process; however, in others, it is very important in understanding and interpreting the performance of the client on the various test measures. For example, prior education would be a consideration in the assessment of a child with language learning disabilities, because the examiner needs to be aware of the child's success or lack of success in the academic environment (Kamhi, 1998; Leonard, 1998). Similarly, it is important to know the educational level of the adult who presents with aphasia (Rosenbeck et al., 1989) when evaluating test performance. The occupation of a client can also be an important concern, because education and vocational status are closely related. Recommendations may need to be made regarding the continuation of employment or aspirations for future vocational opportunities, and those recommendations may depend in large part on the communication skills of the client and the potential for improvement with treatment.

Emotional/Social Status

Similar to observations made in other subsections of the case history, emotional/social status may or may not be an important concern in the communication assessment. Peterson and Marquardt (1990) suggest that the examiner question the client or caregiver in this regard, and they list a number of behavioral characteristics that may be explored.

For example, are there feelings and attitudes that the client expresses regarding the communication disorder? In some cases, there are no negative feelings or attitudes associated with the communication disorder; in others, the client has developed negative feelings and attitudes that are part of the communication disorder. Assessment for persons with suspected fluency disorders often include interview and the use of assessment measures to examine the client's attitudes toward the disorder (Blood, 1998). Some voice disorders, as Stemple (1998) has noted, may also stem from personality-related causes, and the collection of interpersonal data is most important in forming a diagnosis. As social beings, we interact daily with a diverse group of people. Interpersonal skills or how we adjust to others across various situational contexts is very important. Problems in interpersonal adjustment can be a consideration in diagnosis.

Family Dynamics

Generally, the client is a member of some familial unit, and the communication disorder has some perceived impact on other family members. Hubbell (1981) has pointed out that a central theme in family systems theory is the concept of family homeostasis. That is, families seek a state of balance among members. If a family member engages in behavior that is different from the expected family norm, other family members react in an effort to modify the unwanted behavior. Conversely, positive changes in the behavior of a family member can influence the other family members. Hubbell points out that observations of a child during the stages of language development is a good example of positive change, because family members alter their style of communicative interactions in response to the changes that the child displays. Suffice to say that a communication disorder affects the family regardless of whether the patient is a child or adult. Caregivers and spouses have certain perceptions and concerns that they often express to the examiner. Such issues should be noted by the examiner and appropriate feedback provided when necessary.

Cultural variation is another important factor that needs to be considered when planning and conducting an assessment. Modern American society comprises a diverse group of individuals who may differ with respect to cultural, ethnic, religious, and geographic backgrounds (Anderson, 1991). Clinicians need to be aware of such differences when dealing with expressed matters or providing information to concerned family members. Hegde (1996) stressed the fact that variables related to one's cultural, ethnic, social, and personal preferences need to be taken into account, because they can influence the outcome of a diagnostic assessment. For example, practitioners need to be aware of differences in the prevalence of communication disorders and medical conditions across different cultural groups. They must also take into account the beliefs and attitudes that a person has regarding communication and communication disorders, because these variables can affect assessment recommendations. It is also important to identify any cultural barriers that may limit a person's access to recommended therapeutic services. Finally, and most important, the examiner needs to demonstrate a respect and sensitivity for a client's culture and the ways in which it may influence the outcome of a diagnostic assessment.

Other Relevant Information

During the course of the evaluation, the client or caregiver may offer additional information that may or may not be relevant to the assessment. Family relationships, marital problems, and health issues are some concerns that may be discussed by the family or caregiver. The examiner can collect such information but must decide if it is relevant to the diagnostic evaluation and is to be reported. That is, are there reported factors that are germane to understanding the communication disorder, or are they simply statements that have no bearing on the assessment? The examiner must use professional judgment to identify variables important in the diagnosis and disregard those that are not relevant.

Summary

The taking of a case history provides an often necessary context to understand the communication disorder and its impact on the client. The information collected varies as a function of the client and the communication and related disorder. The history is not just a compilation of facts, but an account of the client's disorder and other related information. The examiner must skillfully guide the client or caregiver through discussion by asking relevant questions, providing opportunities for client or caregiver discussion, and furnishing appropriate feedback. The examiner must then interpret the information and use professional judgment to decide which data accurately describe the client, the communication and related disorder, and any intervening variables (Shprintzen, 1997).

Process Variable: Tests and Measurements

After the collection of case history information, a test battery is usually administered to the client. Cartwright (1993) wrote that assessing client performance and establishing the appropriate diagnosis is a composite of three variables. First, the practitioner must select the appropriate measurement tools. When discussing measurement tools, we frequently think of only paper and pencil tests that are available for diagnostic purposes; however, in some cases, instrumentation is used to measure various acoustic or physiological parameters of interest. In other cases, nonstandardized tasks are used to examine client performance. Second, the clinician must be knowledgeable of the test instruments and instrumentation and well versed in the administration and use of them. Because a diagnosis is to be made, it is imperative that tests and instrumental measurements are administered in a standard and reliable manner. Finally, the practitioner must be able to interpret the results of the test instruments that have been administered. It is underscored here and elsewhere in the chapter that the professional judgment and expertise of the evaluator is extremely important, because a clinical decision needs to be made. Although we often conceptualize the testing portion of the assessment as a uniform entity, it is important to remember the different aspects of assessment, because different skills come into play. Moreover, it is the client's disorder that dictates the need for specific tests or instrumental assessment. It should be stressed that sensitivity to cultural issues is also important in the selection of assessment materials and tests. Because the development of our assessment tools is generally based on the dominant white middle-class society, adjustments may need to be made that are consistent with the client's cultural, ethnic, religious, and geographic background.

Standardized Tests

Although standardized tests have been subject to criticism, clinicians frequently use such tests when conducting diagnostic evaluations (Hegde, 1996). Standardized tests have been developed to allow comparison between an individual and some normative sample. Underlying this position is the fact that a standardized test actually evaluates the behaviors of interest in a consistent manner. For example, a test of expressive vocabulary is expected to furnish the examiner with accurate information about an aspect of the client's expressive language skills. In addition, the test is expected to provide consistent results with repeated use of the measure. Sometimes we tend to gloss over these psychometric variables as consumers of such tests, but test validity and reliability are very important considerations in a profession that has experienced tremendous growth in test development.

The practitioner must be a careful consumer, because decisions regarding the existence of a disorder are generally based on the results of normative referenced standardized tests (Merrell & Plante, 1997). Clinicians are strongly urged to examine the psychometric characteristics of tests before purchasing them for use. Hutchinson (1996) provides an excellent account of the psychometric characteristics of tests and includes a series of 20 questions that practitioners may use in evaluating a test. The discussion encompasses processes, procedures, and theory of test development in terms that can be understood by persons who are unfamiliar with test construction and psychometric variables.

McCauley and Swisher (1984a) discuss the concepts of validity and reliability and how they should be conceptualized when examining communication disorder tests. The authors state that test validity is a composite of appropriate test construction and test appraisal. The test developer attempts to select a pool of items that provide an adequate sample of the behaviors of interest. When selecting a test for purchase, the clinician should peruse the test development section of the manual critically to examine the measures of validity that have been carried out.

Generally, there are three types of validity relevant to test development: construct, content, and criterion-related. Construct validity examines the degree to which the test actually measures the theoretical construct underlying the test. For example, if a theoretical construct claims that the development of receptive vocabulary increases as the child develops, we would expect that vocabulary test scores would improve with age, and normative data would be expected to demonstrate such a trend. McCauley and Swisher point out that construct validity is difficult to establish, because it is very subjective in nature.

Content validity is frequently measured by having individuals with expertise in the area of assessment inspect the items that compose the test. Judgments or ratings are provided. An author who developed a new test for aphasia might assemble a panel of clinicians with expertise in the area of adult language disorders. The panel members would inspect each item and judge or rate the appropriateness of each in assessing behaviors that are characteristic of aphasia.

Criterion-related validity provides a gauge of the relationship of the test to other measures that purport to measure the same behavior. Criterion-related validity includes both concurrent validity and predictive validity. Concurrent validity is frequently assessed by comparing the test takers' scores with those of some criterion variable. An indirect way of establishing concurrent validity would be to compare the performance of a group of test takers on a test in question with their performance on another test that had already undergone validity studies, then establish congruence between measures. Predictive validity is estimated by determining if performance on the test predicts future performance on a criterion standard. That is, what is the predictive relationship of the test with some measure that will be used to assess the same behaviors in the future? For example, a test developer might determine how well his or her test predicts future performance on an established test that will also be administered to the normative population.

Reliability is another critical psychometric variable that the clinician needs to consider carefully in test selection (Cartwright, 1993; Hegde, 1996; McCauley & Swisher, 1984a). A reliable test consistently measures what it is supposed to measure. An unreliable test would impinge on validity, because it would not provide consistent assessment of what it was designed to measure. Generally, test developers assess test-retest reliability and interexaminer reliability and report the data in the test manual. Test-retest reliability is a measure of the consistency of results across repeated administrations of the test. A reliable test of phonology would yield similar scores across subjects with repeated administration. That is, one would not expect a significant change in phonological skills over a short period of time. A test that produced extremely fluctuating scores would not be a reliable measure of phonological skills. A test must also be designed to enable reliable administration and scoring among examiners. Interexaminer reliability assesses the stability of scores for subjects across examiners. If interexaminer reliability were not satisfactory, the results of the test would differ as a function of the examiner. Most tests in speech-language pathology can be scored reliably because the items and scoring system can be used by most practitioners; however, there are tests that use multidimensional scoring systems that require extensive training to establish and maintain interexaminer reliability (Porch, 1971).

In addition to validity and reliability, the practitioner also needs to be cognizant of the normative test sample and the scores used in the interpretation of the test. The normative sample consists of the group of individuals who have been tested and their data summarized statistically to allow comparisons between a specific person and the normative group. The test manual should contain information regarding the selection characteristics of the normative group. Selection variables such as age, sex, and socioeconomic status should be reviewed before using a test. Often, practitioners overlook the information and simply use the normative data. Because a comparison is to be made, the practitioner needs to be confident that the client being tested possesses the same selection characteristics of the normative sample.

Concern for normative sample characteristics is very important when dealing with multicultural populations. Because our assessment tools are generally based on white middle-class society, adjustments may need to be made that are consistent with the client's background. Battle (1998) urges extreme caution in using normative data for multicultural populations, because the normative sample generally consists of mainstream cultures; however, developing normative data for various multicultural populations is often not feasible because of the cost involved. It is to be noted that the normative sample of a test is an important concern in selecting or not selecting a particular test.

After the test has been administered, the person's performance or raw score is converted to some type of numerical score, so that statistical comparison with the normative sample may be made. The three most common types of derived scores are age-equivalent scores, percentile scores, and standard scores (Cartwright, 1993). McCauley and Swisher (1984a) state that the derived scores differ with respect to the information that they provide; consequently, there are a number of issues that need to be considered carefully with the different scoring systems. Practitioners should be aware of this when making decisions regarding the presence or absence of a communication or related disorder.

Age-equivalent scores are frequently used to report certain behaviors or skills that change as a function of age during development. The major advantage of this type of score is that parents and professionals from other disciplines can readily understand it. When a practitioner reviews a child's performance on a test and indicates that the age-equivalent score was 6 years, 7 months, one can easily comprehend the comparison; however, there are certain disadvantages to using age-equivalent scores. Cartwright (1993) points out that age-equivalent scores provide no real basis for analyzing a child's performance in relation to some peer group. A depressed age-equivalent score does not necessarily mean that a child's performance is depressed, but may reflect normal variation in peer achievement. The use of age-equivalent scores is not a satisfactory means of establishing normative performance and should be used only in combination with other types of test scores (McCauley & Swisher, 1984b).

A percentile score allows comparison of the person's test performance with normative scores that fall higher and lower than the obtained score value. For example, a percentile score of 65 indicates that 35% of the normative population received higher scores, whereas 65% received similar or lower scores. McCauley and Swisher (1984a) state that percentile scores can be easily interpreted by test examiners; however, there are also certain problems associated with the use of such score comparisons. One such problem is that small differences at the lower end of the scale (<10) or the higher end of the scale (>90) can actually represent very large differences in raw score values. This occurs because most individuals receive scores within the range of average, so there is not a widespread dispersion of raw score values.

The most preferred score from an interpretive viewpoint is the standard score. Standard scores enable the examiner to understand a test score as it compares with the average normative score and the dispersion or deviation from the average score. The theoretical normal distribution is the basis for standard score interpretation. Often practitioners shy away from the use of statistical-type measurement, but standard scores are equal measurement units and can be managed through mathematical means. The use of standard scores enables accurate comparison between the test taker and the normative group. The most commonly used type of standard score is the z score. The mean value for the z distribution is 0, and the standard deviation is 1. A score within the values of 1.00 and –1.00 is in the range of average performance on the test in question. A score higher than 1.00 is above average, just as a score lower than –1.00 is below average. Various regulatory agencies have begun to set certain standard score values to establish client selection criteria for treatment; a practice that has questionable value in determining which clients receive services (Reed, 1994).

Criterion-Referenced Tests

Although most tests in speech-language pathology are normative referenced, there are tests that provide a criterion-referenced account of performance. A criterion-referenced test is an instrument that has been designed to assess a set of skills without normative comparison. The test is an assessment of the client's acquisition of the skills in question to identify which skills have been mastered and which have not. McCauley (1996) provided a cogent discussion of the characteristics of criterion-referenced tests. She explained that such testing is designed to identify particular levels of student performance across a specific domain of related skills. The items selected for testing purposes purport to assess the content domain; the performance of an individual with such measures can be specified by simply using the obtained raw score. The Basic Concept Inventory (Engelmann, 1967) is an example of a criterion-referenced measure. The author assembled a set of items that were determined to be important linguistic concepts necessary for success in first grade. The test is administered, and those items problematic for a particular client are identified as potential targets for treatment.

Summary

Normative tests are used quite extensively to assess various speech, language, and related behaviors. As consumers of such tests, practitioners should be well versed in the construction, development, administration, and interpretation of such measures. There are a number of important concerns that one needs to consider when using a particular measure. Shipley and McAfee (1992), like Hutchinson (1996), stress the importance of knowing the characteristics of tests, and the authors developed a checklist that practitioners may use to evaluate a test for possible selection. In addition, the American Psychological Association has published the *Code of Fair Testing Practices in Education* (1988). This is a publication that provides information on all aspects of test development and use. In addition to normative measures, there are also criterion-referenced tests. The purpose of these measures is to evaluate a set of skills that have been determined to be within the developmental level of a specific group of individuals. Different types of tests may be used in the assessment process; consequently, the practitioner must be aware of the advantages and disadvantages of each test.

Instrumental Measurement Parameters of Speech and Related Disorders

In addition to the use of normative and criterion-referenced tests, instrumentation may be used to collect acoustic and physiological data that can be used to identify certain features of a particular disorder. Baken (1987) feels that instrumental assessment improves the exactness of the diagnostic findings, facilitates the evaluation of therapeutic intervention, and furnishes objective indices of behavior. Generally, measurement is conducted with sophisticated equipment; however, there are also very simple devices that can be constructed to estimate various acoustic or physiological parameters (Hixon et al., 1982; Mueller et al., 1979). For example, aerodynamic assessment is a physiological study method that examines air pressure, airflow, and air volume within the vocal tract. Such study methods are often used with clients who have a suspected problem with velopharyngeal closure during speech (Moon, 1993). Measurement of oral pressure sounds, such as plosives, fricatives, and affricates, would typically show an expected pattern of oral pressure in the absence of nasal airflow. A pattern of reduced oral pressure and the presence of nasal airflow would suggest that velopharyngeal closure for speech is deficient. The performance data would be used in conjunction with the perceptual observations of the examiner and additional measurement techniques to diagnose the problem.

The advent of computers and the overall improvement in instrumentation have allowed the practitioner to quantify various speech dimensions and study the results in relation to perceptual observations (McGuire, 1995). Related disorders, such as dysphagia, are also subject to instrumental analysis, because all aspects of the swallowing process cannot be studied through behavioral observation exclusively (Logemann, 1998). Shuster (1993) discussed the various measurement parameters and stated that:

TABLE 1.3   A summary of physiological and acoustic measurement parameters

Physiological measures
   Air pressure
   Airflow
   Air volume
   Movement studies
Acoustic measures
   Frequency
   Intensity
   Time

Speech and speech disorders are usually described three ways: acoustically, physiologically, and perceptually. Physiological phonetics is defined as the study of sound production and movements of the body that produce sounds; acoustic phonetics is defined as the study of the sound waves that are produced as speech; and perceptual phonetics is the study of the auditory cues that allow us to identify and discriminate speech (p. 26).

Physiological Measures: Air Pressure, Airflow, and Air Volume

A listing of the various measurement parameters according to study method is listed in Table 1.3. Aerodynamic assessment is a physiological study method that examines air pressure, airflow, and air volume within the vocal tract. Air pressure, airflow, and air volume are inextricably related, and evaluation of one or more of the parameters is often used in a speech assessment. Baken (1987) indicated that the sounds of the language are generated through use of air pressure produced by the respiratory system, and the study of pressure at different locations of the vocal tract can be very useful. For example, stops are made with a complete closure of the vocal tract and then a release of the closure. Air pressure is built up behind the constriction and then quickly released into the atmosphere (Kent & Read, 1992). The buildup of air pressure within the vocal tract can be measured with instrumentation and the values compared with normative data (Baken, 1987; Kent, 1994).

A typical procedure to measure intraoral pressure would require the placement of a pressure-sensing tube in the mouth situated perpendicular and behind the sound constriction. The pressure fluctuations are collected and then channeled to a differential pressure transducer that converts the pressure into electrical energy. The electrical energy is then fed into a computer for display and analysis. Air pressure is generally measured in centimeters of water pressure; consequently, a pressure value of 8 cm H_2O means that the measured pressure would elevate a column of water 8 centimeters in height.

Airflow is the amount of air that moves through a specified area in a particular unit of time. When a gas such as air is driven from a region of higher pressure to a region of lower pressure, the flow of gas can be measured. Baken (1987) pointed out that fluctuations in airflow reflect the different variations in consonant and vowel productions. Moreover, the study of airflow can assist in diagnosis, be used as a measure to evaluate change during treatment, and function as a biofeedback technique to patients with certain speech disorders. Oral airflow measurements may be made during vowel and consonant productions, or samples of nasal airflow may be obtained during speech tasks. There are a number of instrumental methods, but airflow is generally measured via a collection device known as a *pneumotachograph*, which is attached to a face mask. The pneumotachograph contains a fine wire-mesh screen that serves as a resistance to airflow. The resistance or pressure drop across the screen is proportional to the airflow through it. The pressure drop is transferred to a differential pressure transducer, which converts the pressure into electrical energy. The electrical energy is transformed by a computer for display and analysis. Measures of airflow are typically expressed in milliliters or liters of air per second, and normative data have been obtained for both children and adults. In some cases, air pressure and airflow are collected simultaneously to evaluate certain speech disorders.

The final aerodynamic parameter is that of air volume, or the amount of air that is expended by an individual for a particular nonspeech or speech task (Shuster, 1993). Wet and dry spirometers are reliable instruments that can be used to measure various lung volumes, such as vital capacity. Vital capacity is the maximum amount of air expelled after a maximum inspiration of air, and it varies as a function of sex, body size, and breathing postures. Baken (1987) affirmed the reliability of the spirometer for nonspeech volume measurement but warned that the instrumentation is not well suited for measuring small, fast-changing volumes that occur during speech production. Individuals using the instrumentation for speech volume determination must exercise caution.

Two measures of volume often used in the study of speech are articulatory volume and phonatory volume. Articulatory volume is the volume of air used in the production of individual sounds or syllables. An estimate of volume can be obtained by having a person repeat a predetermined test stimulus on a single breath and measuring the total air volume with a spirometer. Phonatory volume is evaluated by having the client take a maximum inhalation and then phonate as long as possible, keeping pitch and loudness constant. Measurements are taken with a spirometer or pneumotachograph integrator system. Normative data exist for both volume indices and can be used for clients with disorders of phonation or articulation. Figure 1.1 shows an aerodynamic assessment of oral air pressure and nasal airflow. A tube is placed in the oral cavity to sense pressure, and a mask attached to a pneumotachograph measures nasal airflow.

Physiological Measures: Movement Studies

There have been a number of techniques developed that can be used to study the movements of the vocal tract during both speech and nonspeech tasks (Baken, 1987; Logemann, 1998; Shuster, 1993). Although

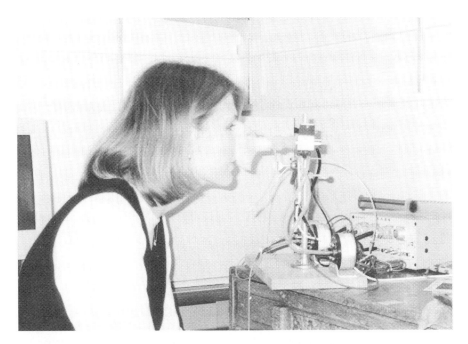

FIGURE 1.1   *An assessment of oral air pressure and nasal airflow.*

somewhat arbitrary, it is useful to dichotomize techniques into indirect and direct study methods. Indirect study methods provide an inferential measure of physiology, whereas direct study methods furnish a direct visualization of the physiology in question.

One of the most frequently used indirect methods is that of electromyography, or the measurement of muscle action potential from muscles used in speech production (Moon, 1993). Electrodes are placed on muscle surfaces or inserted into the muscle to record muscle action potential. The electrical energy associated with muscle contraction is directed to an amplifier, which amplifies the energy so that it can be displayed for analysis. Electromyography is used extensively in speech research and can also be used in the diagnosis of motor speech disorders and biofeedback treatment studies (Denny & Smith, 1992; Duffy, 1995). Although a practitioner might not use electromyography for diagnosis, it is entirely likely that case history information might include such data for a client with a suspect neurophysiologic problem.

Electropalatography is a technology that is capable of recording linguapalatal contacts during speech production. The person is fitted with a custom-made palatal appliance containing electrodes. The tongue comes in contact with the electrodes, and the configuration during the production of a sound is captured. Dagenais (1995) stated that the major advantage of electropalatography is that it "provides a dynamic, real-time, visual presentation of articulatory gestures that are normally not seen" (p. 305). Furthermore, acoustic and perceptual measures do not provide an accurate description of the correct/incorrect articulatory gestures that are used by a particular speaker. There is definitely merit in using electropalatography; however, the instrumentation requires the design of a custom palatal appliance, a drawback that prohibits widescale use in diagnosis.

Movement of the articulators can also be studied through the use of various movement transduction instruments (Baken, 1987). The range and force of articulatory movements—of the lips and jaw, for example—can be measured through the use of strain-gauge systems. Rigid wires, attached to a strain gauge, are positioned to certain articulators, such as the lips. A person is then instructed to carry out a movement task involving the lips. The displacements of the upper and lower lips are sensed by the strain gauge, which creates an electrical voltage proportional to the detected movement. The output is then recorded for study purposes. Electromagnetic transduction is an investigative procedure used for recording articulatory movements. Baken (1987) points out that the methodology was originally developed for measuring movement of the chest wall, but it has also been used to track other movements, such as jaw and tongue motion. The instrumentation consists of a generator coil and sensor coils, which create a magnetic field. Change in movement is a function of the distance between the generator coil and the sensor coils. As distance changes between the generator and sensor coils, electrical voltage varies and furnishes data regarding the timing, coordination, and amount of movement studied.

Direct visualization of the vocal tract is possible through a number of different instrumental approaches that have been used in the study of speech and related disorders, such as dysphagia (Baken, 1987; Logemann, 1998). Endoscopy is a direct technique used to observe vocal tract movement. An endoscope is a telescopic system with appropriate illumination that can be inserted in the vocal tract. An endoscope can be inserted orally, but typically is placed into a naris and positioned to observe velopharyngeal closure during speech, laryngeal structure and function, and pharyngeal phenomena before and after swallowing (Langmore et al., 1988; Logemann, 1998; Moon, 1993). Generally, the endoscope is attached to a video camera so that a visual record can be made for assessment purposes.

Ultrasound is an imaging process used to study movement of the oral portion of the vocal tract. High-frequency sound waves are transferred to the body via a transducer that is in contact with a body surface. The transducer contains a crystal that acts to change electrical energy to high-frequency acoustic pulses. The acoustic energy is radiated into the body area of interest. The acoustic pulses are reflected back from the body to the transducer and converted into electrical energy. The signals provide an image of the anatomic area of interest that can be recorded or displayed. Although not used extensively in speech research, it has been used in studies of dysphagia (Shawker et al., 1983).

One of the most frequently used direct visualization procedures is that of radiography (Moon, 1993). The basic principle of radiography is that electrons come in contact with an intensifying screen and cause the screen to emit light. The intensity of the light varies as a function of the number of electrons coming in contact with the screen at any given time. The number of electrodes modulates in relation to the density of the anatomic site being studied. The process has evolved from the use of still radiographs or x-ray films to motion picture recording to videofluoroscopic or video recording of speech and movements of related disorders, such as dysphagia (Logemann, 1998). Such visualization techniques are very important in understanding the physiology of the vocal tract. Additional viewing techniques include computerized tomography and magnetic resonance imaging (MRI). Computerized tomography is a radiographic technique that uses a computer to isolate an anatomic section of interest. A client is generally placed in the supine position, and the x-ray electrons are aimed in a way that detectors can measure the x-ray beam at different points after the beam has passed through the body. The resultant image is that of a particular anatomic structure in the transverse plane. MRI does not use x-ray, but rather sends radio-frequency impulses into the body that interact with hydrogen atoms. Hydrogen nuclei are found in all body tissue that contains water. When stimulated by the magnetic field of the MRI, the hydrogen nuclei become aligned. The alignment of the hydrogen nuclei is altered by the radio-frequency impulses, and as the nuclei return to their natural state, there is a transfer of energy that is detected by a radio receiver. The images are then presented via tomographic sections for view.

Acoustic Study

Acoustics is that part of physics that pertains to the study of sound, and psychoacoustics is the investigation of one's response to sound (Kent & Read, 1992). In the study of speech disorders, we are interested in the physical structure of the sounds of our language, as well as in the perception of those speech sounds. Investigators may study the speech signal with instrumentation that permits measurement of frequency, amplitude, and duration characteristics. In addition, speech may be synthesized through artificial means by manipulating the variables of frequency, amplitude, and duration. Although some current practitioners may not have access to instrumentation for acoustic analysis, the development and use of such equipment continue to increase in the profession (McGuire, 1995; Read et al., 1990). Read et al. (1992) state that current technological advances hold real promise for the development of an expanded acoustic database that may be used in teaching, research, and clinical applications.

Sound spectrography—the measurement of the acoustic signal into its fundamental components—is often used for analysis purposes. A spectrogram is generated and displayed via a video screen, or a hard copy of the data is produced. The usual spectrogram furnishes a display of frequency, intensity, and duration information (Kent & Read, 1992). These data can assist the clinician in the assessment of a client's communication disorder through the collection of information such as formant frequencies, formant transitions, noise spectra, and voice onset time. Figure 1.2 displays a spectrogram showing a series of isolated vowel productions.

Some researchers have used acoustic information as a form of biofeedback to an individual. For example, Shuster et al. (1992) assessed acoustically defective /r/ productions from a person who had not improved his articulation of /r/ after substantial traditional therapy. After assessment, tokens of correct /r/ and incorrect /r/ were shown to the client for visual contrast pur-

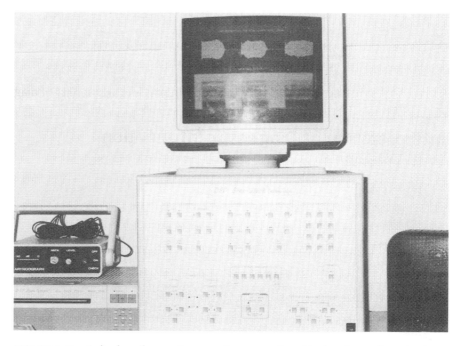

FIGURE 1.2 *A display of a spectrogram shows a series of isolated vowel productions.*

poses. The acoustic contrast was then followed by a production stage in which the client was instructed to observe the computer screen and match correct /r/ target formant patterns with practice productions. The client was successful in using the abstract acoustic information to produce correct /r/ productions. Although this is just one example, there are numerous applications in the literature of acoustic analysis being used in both the assessment and treatment of persons with various speech disorders (McGuire, 1995).

There are also other acoustic measures that are used in the evaluation of different communication disorders. For example, shimmer and jitter are two acoustic parameters that are often assessed with clients who have voice disorders. Shimmer is the measurement of changes in the amplitude of a signal. It is hypothesized that significant variations in the amplitude of fundamental frequency are related to the perceptual identification of hoarseness (Baken, 1987). Jitter is the perturbation or fluctuation in fundamental frequency that occurs during laryngeal vibration (Kent & Read, 1992). As with shimmer, it is thought that extensive variations in fundamental frequency or jitter are correlates of the perceptual dimension of hoarseness.

Summary

Assessment of communication and related disorders may include the use of instrumentation for the purpose of providing objective data. Technological advances have allowed practitioners to measure different acoustic and physiological variables, which are important to the establishment of an accurate diagnosis. For example, direct visualization techniques can show the physiology of both speech and nonspeech gestures used in tasks such as speaking and swallowing. In some cases, the use of objective information acts to supplement perceptual observations, whereas in others, it provides a standard for a diagnosis. Practitioners need to become familiar with instrumentation and the information that it provides, because it is becoming an important part of diagnosis.

Interpretation of Diagnostic Information

After the diagnostic information has been obtained, the clinician must carefully examine the assessment results and interpret them to make the correct diagnosis. This is not just an exercise that involves scoring tests, making normative comparisons, or inspecting some instrumental assessment. It is a mental process that centers on the interpretation of the assessment data in combination with the history information that has been collected. Interpretation leads to the identification of the disorder and recommendations regarding treatment; in some cases, treatment is not feasible for a particular client and is not recommended. These are decisions made by the practitioner after careful scrutiny of the diagnostic data. The point to be made is that it is the practitioner's responsibility to render such clinical decisions based on best practice. Diagnosis is one of those clinical responsibilities that is a function of professional skill and education. The practitioner is not a technician but a professional who has been educated to make such clinical decisions.

Nation and Aram (1982) present a conceptual framework that they recommend to interpret diagnostic findings. Their first recommendation is to study the results of the assessment and the history data, so that the practitioner is aware of all available information. How do these data sets relate to each other? Is there sufficient information, or are there gaps in the data? What are the significant pieces of information that lead to the appropriate conclusions? Does the information confirm the practitioner's clinical hypothesis, or is it necessary to revise the hypothesis in light of the data? To answer these questions, the practitioner must identify the significant aspects of the data and develop the most reasonable explanation. This process requires the practitioner to call on his or her diagnostic knowledge and reasoning powers. Interpretation is a product of the practitioner's education, clinical experience, and familiarity with the current research literature.

After the diagnosis has been made, results and recommendations must be interpreted for the client, caregiver, and other professionals in terms that they can understand rather than in the technical jargon of the profession. This is extremely important for the client who is seeking information and the caregivers who must also understand the diagnosis and its implications. In the case of youngsters or persons with severe disabilities, it is particularly important that the findings be clearly communicated, because significant others must understand the diagnosis and recommendations. For example, if a client was diagnosed with hypernasal speech, the characteristics and physiology of the problem and recommendations would need to be presented in a manner that could be understood by all involved. Similarly, referrals to other professionals must be clearly communicated, because they need to understand the diagnosis and any implications for their professional discipline. What is to be done and why it is necessary to obtain such additional information must be clearly communicated.

The final step in interpretation is the preparation of a written report of the findings and required letters to those who are also involved in providing various types of service to the client. Generally, the report is forwarded to the client, referral source, and any additional entities that have been designated. Like the verbal communication, the written report must be grammatically correct and composed in terms that can be understood by all involved. Other practitioners in the professions may understand the technical jargon, but many who need to read the report do not. The caution to be clear and concise is warranted in the report, because it is the written summary of the case history, testing, and interpretation of the overall assessment. The profession places great emphasis on report writing. A clinical variable used in the evaluation of Clinical Fellows states: "written reports, and letters are always appropriate for the needs of the audience" (ASHA, 1997, p. 95). Hegde (1998) points out that the written report varies in reference to the practice setting and recipients of the report. This means that the practitioner must carefully modify his or her writing to the diagnostic context.

Summary

The interpretation of the diagnostic findings is a challenging task for the practitioner. All pertinent information and test data must carefully be considered before a diagnosis can be made. The practitioner's education, clinical experience, knowledge of the research literature, and reasoning skills come into play. Once the diagnosis has been made, it must be communicated in both verbal and written form to the client, caregivers, and others involved in the client's care.

Professional Judgment

If one reads any text on assessment or has participated in an assessment course, there is generally a series of guidelines that are listed for consideration in the overall scheme of the evaluation process. For example, Bernthal and Bankson (1998) cogently discuss variables that may be factors in the assessment of a phonological disorder. In addition to phonological performance variables, they cite other variables—such as dialect and social-vocational expectations—as potential elements that could come into play in rendering a final diagnosis for a particular client. The point is that despite all the guidelines, education, and experience, the practitioner must interpret the diagnostic data within an internalized investigative process.

A major intellectual tool used in the investigative process is that of professional judgment. One may ponder the legitimacy of such an abstract concept, but the position presented herein is that it is a compilation of the practitioner's education, reasoning skills, and clinical development. Moll (1983) has stressed the position that graduate educational programs need to infuse practitioners with knowledge, skills, and attitudes that will enable them to foster novel and variant use of the current knowledge base. Moreover, as the knowledge base changes through experimental inquiry, practitioners must avail themselves of the new knowledge.

One might reflect on the characteristics that foster professional judgment. As discussed previously, it appears that education and experience are two factors that contribute significantly to professional judgment; however, professional judgment is an ongoing process that reflects the clinical and cognitive growth of the individual. Schon (1983) has stated that practitioners in a profession that is grounded in science must engage in ongoing inquiry because of the diversity of problems facing them. One needs to look at a current problem, such as diagnosis, within an internally developed grid of problem-solving techniques that are part of the practitioner's professional judgment skills. Each new client is envisioned as a problem with certain commonalties and differences in relation to other clients. The practitioner evaluates all pertinent information and performance data to arrive at an appropriate diagnosis.

In this conceptualization, professional judgment would not be static, but rather a dynamic process that changes as a function of lifelong learning and clinical experience. Preprofessional and professional education, continuing education and in-service work, journal/book reading, and professional ethics are key elements in the development of an intellectual framework that nurtures professional judgment. Similarly, clinical experiences with individual clients, clinical work with other colleagues, and interactions with allied professionals are work-related factors that also play a role in the evolution of professional judgment.

Summary

In this chapter, I have presented a general model for the diagnosis of communication and related disorders and discussed its individual components. An underlying theoretical model guides the assessment of clients. Based on the theoretical position, certain information is collected, and tests are administered to furnish pertinent client data. After the collection of the data, the practitioner interprets the findings so that an accurate diagnosis can be made. Interpretation is an important aspect of the diagnostic process and is a reflection of the practitioner's professional judgment. Professional judgment is a mentalistic process that is requisite to diagnosis and integral to the diagnostic process. Furthermore, professional judgment is a composite of many factors and must evolve over time if the practitioner is to meet the continual challenge of accurate diagnosis.

References

American Psychological Association, Joint Committee on Testing Practices. (1988). *Code of fair testing practices in education*. Washington, DC: Author.

American Speech-Language Hearing Association, Clinical Certification Board. (1997). *Membership & certification handbook*. Rockville, MD: Author.

Anderson, N. B. (1991). Understanding cultural diversity. *American Journal of Speech-Language Pathology, 1,* 9–10.

Baken, R. J. (1987). *Clinical measurement of speech and voice*. San Diego: College-Hill Press.

Battle, D. E. (1998). Differential diagnosis of communication disorders in multicultural populations. In B. J. Philips & D. M. Ruscello (Eds.), *Differential diagnosis in speech-language pathology* (pp. 5–44). Boston: Butterworth–Heinemann.

Bernthal, J. E., & Bankson, N. W. (1998). *Articulation and phonological disorders* (4th ed.). Needham Heights, MA: Allyn & Bacon.

Blood, G. W. (1998). Differential diagnosis for fluency disorders. In B. J. Philips & D. M. Ruscello (Eds.), *Differential diagnosis in speech-language pathology* (pp. 159–188). Boston: Butterworth–Heinemann.

Bonem, H. (1994). Attention deficit hyperactivity disorder: A clinical overview. *HearSay, 9,* 5–14.

Camarata, S., & Swisher, L. (1990). A note on intelligence assessment within studies of specific language impairment. *Journal of Speech and Hearing Research, 33,* 205–207.

Campbell, T. F. (1998). Themes in diagnostic decision making. *Seminars in Speech and Language, 19,* 3–6.

Cartwright, L. R. (1993). The challenge of interpreting test scores. *Clinics in Communication Disorders, 3,* 17–25.

Dagenais, P. A. (1995). Electropalatography in the treatment of articulation/phonological disorders. *Journal of Communication Disorders, 28,* 303–330.

Denny, M., & Smith, A. (1992). Gradations in a pattern of neuromuscular activity associated with stuttering. *Journal of Speech and Hearing Research, 35,* 1216–1229.

Deputy, P. N., & Weston, A. D. (1998). A framework for differential diagnosis of phonological disorders. In B. J. Philips & D. M. Ruscello (Eds.), *Differential diagnosis in speech-language pathology* (pp. 113–158). Boston: Butterworth–Heinemann.

Duffy, J. R. (1995). *Motor speech disorders*. St. Louis: Mosby-Year Book, Inc.

Engelmann, S. E. (1967). *The basic concept inventory*. Chicago: Follett Publishing Company.

Hegde, M. N. (1996). *Pocket guide to assessment in speech-language pathology*. San Diego: Singular Publishing Group, Inc.

Hegde, M. N. (1998). *A coursebook on scientific and professional writing for speech-language pathology*. San Diego: Singular Publishing Group, Inc.

Hixon, T. J., Hawley, J. L., & Wilson, K. J. (1982). An around-the-house device for the clinical determination of respiratory driving pressure: A note on making simple even simpler. *Journal of Speech and Hearing Disorders, 47,* 413–415.

Hubbell, R. D. (1981). *Children's language disorders: An integrated approach*. Englewood Cliffs, NJ: Prentice-Hall, Inc.

Hutchinson, T. A. (1996). What to look for in the technical manual: Twenty questions for users. *Language, Speech, and Hearing Services in Schools, 27,* 109–121.

Kamhi, A. (1998). Differential diagnosis of language learning disabilities. In B. J. Philips & D M. Ruscello (Eds.), *Differential diagnosis in speech-language pathology* (pp. 87–112). Boston: Butterworth–Heinemann.

Kent, R. D. (1994). *Reference manual of communicative sciences and disorders.* Austin, TX: Pro-Ed.

Kent, R. D., & Read, C. (1992). *The acoustic analysis of speech.* San Diego: Singular Publishing Group, Inc.

Langmore, S. E., Schatz, K., & Olson, M. (1988). Fiberoptic endoscopic examination of swallowing safety: A new procedure. *Dysphagia, 2,* 216–219.

Leonard, L. B. (1998). *Children with specific language impairment.* Cambridge: MIT Press.

Logemann, J. A. (1998). *Evaluation and treatment of swallowing disorders* (2nd ed.). Austin, TX: Pro-Ed.

McCauley, M. C. (1996). Familiar strangers: Criterion-referenced measures in communication disorders. *Language, Speech, and Hearing Services in Schools, 27,* 122–131.

McCauley, R. J., & Swisher, L. (1984a). Psychometric review of language and articulation tests for preschool children. *Journal of Speech and Hearing Disorders, 49,* 34–42.

McCauley, R. J., & Swisher, L. (1984b). Use and misuse of norm-referenced tests in clinical assessment: A hypothetical case. *Journal of Speech and Hearing Disorders, 49,* 338–348.

McGuire, R. A. (1995). Computer-based instrumentation: Issues in clinical applications. *Language, Speech, and Hearing Services in Schools, 26,* 223–231.

Meitus, I. J. (1983). Approaching the diagnostic process. In I. J. Meitus & B. Weinberg (Eds.), *Diagnosis in speech-language pathology* (pp. 1–30). Baltimore: University Park Press.

Merrell, A. W., & Plante, E. (1997). Norm-referenced test interpretation in the diagnostic process. *Language, Speech, and Hearing Services in Schools, 28,* 50–58.

Moll, K. (1983). Issue II: Graduate education. In N. S. Rees & T. L. Snope (Eds.), *Proceedings of the 1983 conference on undergraduate, graduate, and continuing education* (pp. 25–37). Rockville, MD: American Speech-Language Hearing Association.

Moon, J. B. (1993). Evaluation of velopharyngeal function. In K. T. Moller & C. D. Starr (Eds.), *Cleft palate: Interdisciplinary issues and treatment* (pp. 251–306). Austin, TX: Pro-Ed.

Mueller, P. B., Adams, M., Baehr-Rouse, J., & Boos, D. A. (1979). A tape striation counting method for determining fundamental frequency. *Language, Speech, and Hearing Services in Schools, 10,* 246–248.

Nation, J. E., & Aram, D. M. (1982). The diagnostic process. In N. J. Lass, L. V. McReynolds, J. L. Northern, & D. E. Yoder (Eds.), *Speech, hearing and language* (pp. 443–460). Philadelphia: W. B. Saunders.

Owens, R. Jr. (1984). *Language development: An introduction* (1st ed.). Boston: Allyn & Bacon.

Owens, R. Jr. (1996). *Language development: An introduction* (4th ed.). Boston: Allyn & Bacon.

Peterson, H. A., & Marquardt, T. P. (1990). *Appraisal and diagnosis of speech and language disorders* (2nd ed.). Englewood Cliffs, NJ: Prentice-Hall, Inc.

Porch, B. (1971). *The Porch index of communicative ability.* Palo Alto, CA: Consulting Psychologists Press.

Read C., Buder, E. H., & Kent R. D. (1990). Speech analysis systems: A survey. *Journal of Speech and Hearing Research, 33,* 363–374.

Read, C., Buder, E. H., & Kent, R. D. (1992). Speech analysis systems: An evaluation. *Journal of Speech and Hearing Research, 35,* 314–332.

Reed, V. A. (1994). *An introduction to children with language disorders.* New York: Macmillan College Publishing Company.

Rogers, B., & Campbell, J. (1993). Pediatric and neurodevelopmental evaluation. In J. C. Arvedson & L. Brodsky (Eds.), *Pediatric swallowing and feeding* (pp. 5–52). San Diego: Singular Publishing Group, Inc.

Rosenbeck, J. C., La Pointe, L. L., & Wertz, R. T. (1989). *Aphasia: A clinical approach.* Boston: Little, Brown and Company.

Sackett, D. L., Haynes, R. B., Guyatt, T., & Tugwell, P. (1991). *Clinical epidemiology: A basic science for clinical medicine.* Boston: Little, Brown and Company.

Schery, T. K. (1985). Correlates of language development in language-disordered children. *Journal of Speech and Hearing Disorders, 50,* 73–83.

Schery, T. K., & Garber, A. S. (1998). Differential diagnosis for young children presenting with language delay. In B. J. Philips & D. M. Ruscello (Eds.), *Differential diagnosis in speech-language pathology* (pp. 45–86). Boston: Butterworth–Heinemann.

Schon, D. A. (1983). *The reflective practitioner.* New York: Basic Books, Inc.

Shawker, T. H., Sonies, B. C., Stone, M., & Baum, B. (1983). Real-time ultrasound visualization of tongue movement during swallowing. *Journal of Clinical Ultrasound, 11,* 485–494.

Shaywitz, S. E., Fletcher, J. M., & Shaywitz, B. A. (1994). Issues in the definition and classification of attention deficit disorder. *Topics in Language Disorders, 14,* 1–25.

Shipley, K. G., & McAfee, J. G. (1992). *Assessment in speech-language pathology.* San Diego: Singular Publishing Group, Inc.

Shprintzen, R. J. (1997). *Genetic syndromes and communication disorders.* San Diego: Singular Publishing Group, Inc.

Shriberg, L. D., & Kwiatkowski, J. (1982). Phonological disorders I: A diagnostic classification system. *Journal of Speech and Hearing Disorders, 47,* 226–241.

Shuster, L. I. (1993). Interpretation of speech science measures. *Clinics in Communication Disorders, 3,* 26–35.

Shuster L. I., Ruscello, D. M., & Smith, K. D. (1992). Evoking [r] using visual feedback. *American Journal of Speech-Language Pathology, 1,* 29–34.

Stemple, J. C. (1998). Differential diagnosis of voice pathology. In B. J. Philips & D. M. Ruscello (Eds.), *Differential diagnosis in speech-language pathology* (pp. 189–212). Boston: Butterworth–Heinemann.

Weaver, C. (1993). Understanding and educating students with attention deficit hyperactivity disorder: Toward a system theory and whole language perspective. *American Journal of Speech-Language Pathology, 2,* 79–89.

Yoder, D., & Kent, R. (1988). *Decision making in speech-language pathology.* Philadelphia: Decker.

2

Phonological Assessment
of Child Speech

A. Lynn Williams

The foundation and cornerstone to effective intervention of speech disorders in children is an accurate assessment of the child's sound system. Gierut (1986) claims that treatment "can only be as effective as the assessment is thorough and accurate" (p. 83). Although many tests and analyses have remained standard fare, there have been considerable changes over the years in the way children's speech disorders have been assessed. The introduction of phonological principles from the field of linguistics was responsible for many of these changes.

The main contribution of phonological principles is the focus on identification of *patterns* of sound errors rather than on individual sound misarticulations. Although the terms and concept of "phonology" have existed in our literature since the 1980s, many clinicians continue to express confusion over the use of phonological terms and principles, as well as uncertainty about the benefits of using a phonological approach in their clinical practice. This uncertainty is reflected by Hodson's (1992) estimate that only approximately 10% of practicing clinicians in the United States and Canada incorporate phonological principles in their clinical practices with children who have speech disorders.

Although assessment of children's speech has become more complex in some respects, it has also become more interesting and challenging. Rather than a simple listing of sound errors by position and error (i.e., substitution, omission, distortion, or addition), clinicians are learning to view each child as a unique speaker of a new "exotic" language in which their task is to discover the rules and patterns of that particular sound system. Clinicians are discovering the "order in the disorder" as they try to piece together the puzzle of each child's unique sound system (Grunwell, 1997). As case examples have documented, children with phonological disorders do not comprise a homogenous group of speakers. In fact, speech disorders reflect the diversity of children as active, creative learners of a sound system. The "order in the disorder" illustrates that these different sound systems are indeed rule governed, logical, and predictable. The ability of parents and other familiar listeners to understand the child is due to the predictable, rule-governed nature of the child's system, which allows them to learn the child's rules or to "speak their language." Our goal as speech-language pathologists is to use assessment tools that help us discover the logical rules and patterns that govern the child's unique sound system.

The information presented in this chapter summarizes the continued growth in the clinical application of phonological principles in the assessment of children's speech. This chapter provides a basis for discovering the order in children's speech disorders using three different analyses: two from a traditional relational analysis framework and one from a more current framework that incorporates both relational and independent analyses. The goal of this chapter is to provide specific information on assessing moderate to profound speech disorders in children. Information on assessing milder articulation sound errors is not discussed; nor are developments in phonological theory involving nonlinear phonology. Readers are encouraged to consult books and articles that cover these topics more comprehensively (e.g., Ball & Kent, 1997; Bernhardt & Stoel-Gammon, 1994; Bernthal & Bankson, 1998).

This chapter is organized in three sections. The first section presents a model of speech disorders in children and an assessment framework that follows from that model. The second section includes a discussion of three different analyses in assessing one child's disordered speech. In the third and final section, reference information is provided to supplement the assessment of children's speech.

Model of Child Speech Disorders

Defining Speech Disorders

As noted previously, the area of child speech disorders has undergone many changes since the 1980s. These changes are also evident in defining *speech disorders*. The broader term of *speech disorders* is used here to encompass both articulation and phonological disorders, as well as to sidestep the confusion often associated with these two terms. Traditionally, *articulation disorder* has been used to refer to speech disorders that are phonetic, relegated primarily to the peripheral aspects of sound production, and often motor based. The term *phonological disorder* has been used to refer to many of the same children previously described as articulation impaired. With the influence of linguistics, especially the seminal publication of Ingram's (1976) book on phonological disorders in children, speech-language pathologists began to analyze patterns among children's erred sounds that suggested a rule-based problem to their speech disorder. As such, phonological disorders are regarded as phonemic errors that, as Fey (1992) states, involve a "language component that governs the manner in which speech sounds are patterned" (p. 226). The difficulty with these terms, however, is that a given child with a speech disorder may exhibit both articulatory and phonological errors. Further, Elbert (1992) suggests that even a speech disorder that has been diagnosed as "phonological" in nature can also have a phonetic or articulatory component.

For the purposes of this chapter, then, the broader term *speech disorders* is used and encompasses speech errors that can be phonetic, phonemic, or both. This term acknowledges the interrelated and interdependent nature of articulation and phonology. It credits a child's acquisition of a complete sound system that includes an inventory of sounds that are used contrastively to signal meaning differences, a set of rules that specify the permissible combinations of sounds and distribution of sounds in the language, and the processes involved in the planning and execution of motor sequences of the peripheral speech mechanism to produce speech sounds. As such, speech disorders encompass errored speech that arises from a peripheral or central level, or both, because a problem in the central, cognitive-phonological processing level would impact the peripheral level of sound production.

Nature of Assessment

According to Grunwell (1997), a phonological analysis is primarily concerned with *identifying, describing,* and *classifying* sound differences in an individual's speech that signal meaning differences. She suggests that there are three key concepts of a phonological analysis: system, structure, and stability.

System includes a set or inventory of different sounds produced by the speaker. A system includes sounds that have a contrastive function, which serves to make each sound phonetically distinct from other sounds. Further, groups of sounds are related to each other in terms of shared properties or characteristics. Sounds can be contrastive, and therefore phonetically distinct, on the basis of three broad characteristics: place, voice, and manner. An adequate phonological system operates such that there is symmetry as in the sound systems of natural languages of the world. This indicates that the sounds are contrastive in place, voice, and manner and function to signal differences in meaning. Further, it is symmetrical because the sounds function contrastively in all word positions (i.e., initial, medial, and final).

Structure refers to the rules and organization of the sound system. The structure of a sound system specifies the distribution and combination of sounds in a language. For example, the sound rules of English specify that the velar nasal [ŋ] cannot occur word-initially and that only certain consonant combinations are permissible (e.g., [pl, bl, kl, gl] are permissible, but not *[tl, dl]).

Stability refers to the predictability of the speaker's systemic and structural patterns or organization of their sound system. The inventory of sounds (system) and the rules that govern the distribution and combination of sounds (structure) provide the organization and therefore predictability of a "phonology."

These three concepts provide a foundation for examining different assessment frameworks used to analyze children's speech disorders. Two additional concepts are important in discussing frameworks for phonological analyses. These are relational and independent analyses.

A relational analysis is one in which the child's productions are compared on a one-to-one basis with the adult standard. Differences between the two productions are then described in terms of substitutions, omissions, distortions, and additions, or, lately, in terms of phonological processes. A relational analysis, then, provides a description of the child's speech *in relation* to the adult sound system. Further, because a relational analysis describes only the sounds produced in error, it is also referred to as an *error analysis* of the child's speech.

Child phonologists have begun to incorporate independent analyses of children's speech (Stoel-Gammon, 1987; Williams, 1993). An independent analysis examines a child's sound system *independently* of the adult sound system. The child's speech is described as a unique, independent, self-contained sound system. As such, no comparisons are made between the child and adult productions. The analysis describes what sounds the child produces, regardless of accuracy relative to the adult target. This is reported in terms of a phonetic sound inventory. An independent analysis also determines the child's syllable structure and distribution of sounds. Notice that the independent analysis describes what the child *does* rather than what the child *does not* do relative to the adult target. This is in direct contrast to the error descriptions of the relational analysis.

Final issues that must also be considered include the type and length of sample obtained for the analysis, phonetic transcription of the sample, and the severity of the child's speech disorder. The sample on which a phonological analysis is based generally involves a sound inventory test or pattern test. Regardless of the type of test, both involve single-word elicitations that sample all English phonemes in all word positions and, in the case of the pattern test, include opportunities to elicit commonly occurring phonological error patterns. Some analyses, such as the Natural Process Analysis (Shriberg & Kwiatkowski, 1980) and the Phonological Assessment of Child Speech (Grunwell, 1985) do not include a set number of elicitation items. Rather, these tests elicit a conversational sample and recommend that assessment be based on a minimum sample of 100–250 words. Still, other analyses, such as the assessment of productive phonological knowledge (Gierut, 1986), use a 256-item single-word protocol that samples all English phonemes a minimum of five times in each word position and elicit potential minimal pairs and morphophonemic alternations.

Regardless of the type of sample elicited, whole-word phonetic transcription must be completed on all the child's responses to complete a phonological analysis. Whole-word transcription provides additional information needed to determine if a child's productions are influenced by other sounds within the same word. Whole-word transcription also allows the clinician to examine consistency of consonant production that would not be possible in sound inventory tests that only examine each consonant once in each word position.

Finally, the severity of the child's speech disorder, and thus his or her level of intelligibility, influences the type of analysis that is most appropriate for a given child. For mild to moderate speech disorders, a relational analysis may be sufficient. A sound inventory test accompanied with a conversational speech sample provides information on the sound(s) in error and the child's intelligibility in connected speech. For more involved disorders that range from severe to profound, both independent and relational analyses are necessary to provide the additional information needed to adequately describe the child's sound system, as well as to design appropriate intervention. For these children, the speech-language pathologist needs to rely more on single-word elicited tests or speech samples, preferably 150–200 words, and use conversational samples as a supplement given the child's limited intelligibility, particularly in unknown contexts.

Two Different Frameworks for Analyzing Speech Sound Disorders

In this section, two different frameworks are presented for analyzing disordered speech. Using these two frameworks—relational analysis and independent analysis—three different analyses are compared using a speech sample from one child. These analyses are place-voice-manner (PVM) analysis (a relational analysis), phonological process analysis (a relational analysis), and systemic phonological analysis (a relational + independent analysis).

Some analyses are more appropriate for children who exhibit mild to moderate speech disorders, whereas other analyses are more appropriate for children who exhibit severe to profound speech disorders. Generally, as noted previously, relational analyses that are based on shorter samples and conversational speech are more appropriate for less severely disordered sound systems. For more involved sound systems, relational and independent analyses, which are based on longer samples of elicited words, are more appropriate.

To illustrate the three different analyses in this chapter, a short data sample from one child, Cameron, is used. Cameron is a 4-year, 10-month-old boy who exhibited a severe phonological disorder. Whole-word transcriptions are provided in Table 2.1 from his single-word responses to the Goldman-Fristoe Test of Articulation (Goldman & Fristoe, 1986).

Relational Analysis

Recall that a relational analysis describes the child's error productions in relation to the adult model. As such, it is also referred to as an *error analysis*. There are several types of analyses within the relational analysis framework, including a traditional substitutions, omissions, distortions, and additions analysis; distinctive feature analysis; PVM analysis; and a phonological process analysis. The latter two analyses are described in this chapter for two reasons. First, phonological process analyses are commonly used tools of assessment. This is due in large part to their "user-friendly" terminology, or labels, which are used to describe com-

TABLE 2.1 Cameron's single-word responses on the *Goldman-Fristoe Test of Articulation*

Target word	Cameron's production	Target word	Cameron's production
house	haʊs	pencils	p˭ɪʔsːʊlz
telephone	dɑfon	that	dæʔ
cup	dʌʔ	carrot	sɛrᵊɪʔs
gun	dʌm	orange	orəɪz
knife	naɪ	bathtub	bæʔːt˭ʌb
window	wɛo	bath	bæʔ
wagon	wædən	thumb	fʌm
wheel	wɪl	finger	fiəʔɚ
chicken	sɪʔən	ring	wĩ
zipper	sɪpɚ	jumping	dʌ̃pɪŋ
scissors	sɪʔɚs	pajamas	θɑmɪð
duck	dʌʔ	plane	fen
yellow	jəʔo	blue	bu
vacuum	bæʔjʊm	brush	fʌᵊ
matches	mæʔɪz	drum	fʌm
lamp	jæp	flag	fæː
shovel	ʃʌʔo	Santa Claus	θæᵊθɑð
car	sar	Christmas tree	trɪθtri
rabbit	ræʔɪʔ	squirrel	traʊl
fishing	fɪsɪŋ	sleeping	fipi
church	ʃɝ˙ts	bed	bɛ
feather	fɛʔɚ	stove	toː

mon error patterns in children's speech. The widespread use and availability of commercial tests of phonological process analyses have also contributed to their frequent use.

Second, phonological process analysis and the PVM analysis were selected because they yield similar results. These two analyses are similar because phonological processes, *in general*, only change one aspect of consonant production—that is, place, voice, or manner of production. By comparing these two analyses, the reader will notice the similarity in phonological descriptions and the ease and use of completing the PVM analysis.

Phonological Process Analysis
There are a number of commercial tests available using a phonological process approach to assess disordered speech. Although the tests vary in the type of sample obtained and the number of processes used to label the child's error patterns, the results are comparable across tests. Dunn

(1982) compared several commercial tests to each other and to an informal phonological process analysis in describing the speech of one child. She found that the Assessment of Phonological Processes (Hodson, 1980) was better than the other tests in identifying the child's error patterns; however, none identified as many patterns as the informal phonological process that was independent of any of the commercial forms.

Edwards (1994) reviewed several current commercial tests of phonological processes and reported that there are some advantages to using an informal analysis that are independent of a closed set of processes for any particular process analysis. She suggested some guidelines for using a nonstandardized phonological process analysis. These included using a representative speech sample of 50–100 words and completing whole-word phonetic transcriptions. Elbert and Gierut (1986) also described a procedure for completing a nonstandardized phonological process analysis. Their example was based on whole-word transcriptions from the Goldman-Fristoe Test of Articulation. Given this, the following phonological process analysis does not use the procedures of any one commercial test, but incorporates general procedures common to all such tests.

Before beginning the phonological process analysis, review the list of common phonological processes provided in Table 2.2. These processes are compiled from phonological processes common to many commercial tests, but are not tied to any one published test. The processes are listed according to syllable structure and sound simplification processes. Syllable structure processes are deletion errors, whereas sound simplification processes include substitution or assimilation sound pattern changes.

You may find that there is more than one phonological process that can be used to label an error. For example, a child's production of [ʃo] for [so] ("sew") can be labeled as *backing* or *palatalization*. Both processes are correct. Your goal, however, in completing a phonological process analysis is to provide the most accurate and best description possible of the child's speech. Palatalization provides a more precise description of what the child is doing rather than the broader and more vague label of backing.

Finally, each phonological process *generally* changes one aspect of consonant production—that is, place, voice, or manner. As a consequence, one sound error may involve several different phonological processes. When this occurs, phonological processes must be applied in a sequential manner to account for all the sound changes that occurred relevant to the adult target. The sequential application of processes is referred to as *process ordering* (Edwards, 1992).

To illustrate process ordering, we can examine a child's production of [dɪʃ] for [fɪʃ] ("fish"). The first sound error is d/f, which involves changes in place, voice, and manner. To account for all these changes, phonological processes are applied in a sequential manner. The order of application in this example is arbitrary. If place is changed first, all other aspects remain constant. That is, target [f] → [s]. Only place changed; voicing and manner stay the same. This change is labeled *apicalization*. To change manner, you would have [s] → [t]. Here, place and voicing are the same, and only manner changed. This change is stopping. Finally, voicing is changed from [t] → [d] by applying the process of prevocalic

TABLE 2.2 List of common phonological processes

Type	Description	Example
Structural processes (deletion processes)		
Final consonant deletion (FCD)	Deletion of a consonant at the end of a word	hot [hɑ]
Initial consonant deletion (ICD)	Deletion of a consonant at the beginning of a word	hot [ɑt]
Cluster reduction (CR)	Deletion of one or more consonants in a consonant cluster	stop [tɑp]; squirrel [kɝl]
Weak syllable deletion (WSD)	Deletion of an unstressed syllable	telephone [tɛfon]
Consonant deletion (CD)	Deletion of an intervocalic consonant	Santa [sæə]
Simplification processes (substitution processes)		
Stopping (ST)	Substitution of a stop for an affricate or fricative	cheese [tiz]; soap [top]
Fronting (FR)	Substitution of an alveolar for a palatal or velar	ship [sɪp]; gum [dʌm]
Backing (BA)	Substitution of a velar or palatal for an alveolar	top [kɑp]
Gliding (GL)	Substitution of a glide for a liquid	read [wid]
Vocalization (VO)	Substitution of a vowel for a liquid	scissors [sɪzʊz]; shovel [ʃʌvo]
Denasalization (DN)	Substitution of an oral consonant for a nasal	mop [dɑp]
Deaffrication (DA)	Substitution of a fricative for an affricate	peach [piʃ]
Apicalization (AP)	Substitution of an apical consonant for a labial	bee [di]
Labialization (LAB)	Substitution of a labial consonant for a lingual	thumb [fʌm]
Glottal replacement (GR)	Substitution of a glottal stop for a consonant in the middle or end of a word	coat [koʔ]
Idiosyncratic (ID)	Unusual or atypical substitution	car [sɑr]
Assimilation processes and whole word processes		
Velar assimilation (VA)	Substitution of a velar for a nonvelar when the word contains another velar	cat [kæk]
Labial assimilation (LA)	Substitution of a labial for a nonlabial when the word contains another labial	pot [pɑp]
Nasal assimilation (NA)	Substitution of a nasal for an oral consonant when the word contains another nasal	mop [mɑm]
Prevocalic voicing (PV)	Substitution of a voiced sound for a voiceless when followed by a vowel in the same syllable	chimney [dɪmni]
Devoicing (DV)	Substitution of a voiceless consonant for a voiced	dog [dɑk]; zip [sɪp]
Reduplication (RD)	Duplication of a stressed syllable within a word	bottle [bɑbɑ]
Epenthesis (EP)	Insertion of a sound in a word	athlete [æθəlit]
Metathesis (ME)	Reversal of two adjacent segments within a word	ask [æks]
Coalescence (CO)	Combination of two adjacent sounds resulting in two sounds being substituted with one	sweep [fip]

voicing. Thus, process ordering requires the application of phonological processes in a sequential manner to account for all the sound changes from the adult target until the child's pronunciation is derived. The [dɪʃ] example is illustrated thus:

/fɪʃ/	Adult target
sɪʃ	Apicalization
tɪʃ	Stopping
dɪʃ	Prevocalic voicing
[dɪʃ]	Child's pronunciation

It should be noted that not all sound errors abide by the general principle that each process changes only one aspect of sound production (i.e., place, voice, or manner). For instance, a common substitution error in children's speech is [w] for [l], such as [wɪp] for "lip." The phonological process of gliding accounts for this error efficiently without applying several processes that change place and manner of production. In addition, unusual or atypical substitution patterns do not follow this general principle. For example, a child may exhibit a sound preference for [tʃ] and replace several target sounds with this affricate, including [l, k, s, ʃ]. To capture this atypical error pattern, it is better to label all such substitutions as *idiosyncratic* rather than try to apply numerous phonological processes to account for the unusual error pattern. Not only will it make more sense to do it as such, but the pattern of idiosyncratic [tʃ] production will be revealed in your summary.

With this preface, we are ready to analyze Cameron's speech using a phonological process analysis. The procedures for completing a non-standardized phonological process analysis on Cameron's single-word responses is similar to the procedures described by Elbert and Gierut (1986). The analysis is completed on the speech sample obtained from the Goldman-Fristoe Test of Articulation.

Because the process analysis is a relational analysis, each sound difference produced by the child is examined in relation to the adult target. Therefore, the first step in the analysis is to broadly transcribe the adult target for each test item. This is a procedure used by Edwards (1986), Elbert and Gierut (1986), and Hodson (1986).

After the target has been transcribed, the next step is to list each phonological process that occurs in the child's production. This second step involves "unraveling" Cameron's productions relative to the target by applying the phonological process that best describes his errors in a sequential fashion. This procedure is continued until all processes have been listed to account for the difference between Cameron's production and the adult target.

A couple of examples may help demonstrate this procedure. For "telephone," Cameron produced [dɑfon]. Remember, the first step is to transcribe the word according to the target production. Then processes are applied in a sequential fashion, moving from left to right, until the child's production is obtained.

Step 1:	/tɛləfon/	Adult target
Step 2:	tɛfon	Weak syllable deletion
	dɛfon	Prevocalic voicing
	[dɑfon]	

Another example is Cameron's production of "scissors":

Step 1:	/sIzɚz/	Adult target
Step 2:	sIsɚs	Postvocalic devoicing (2x)
	sItɚs	Stopping
	sIʔɚs	Glottal replacement
	[sIʔɚs]	

There are a couple of interesting differences in the second example from the first. Notice in this example that postvocalic devoicing applied to both [z] productions; thus, it was counted twice. A second difference was the fact that Cameron produced a glottal stop for target [z], which represents a change in all aspects of consonant production—that is, place, voice, and manner. As a consequence, three different processes were required to account for this single error production. Devoicing accounted for the voicing change, stopping accounted for the manner change, and glottal replacement accounted for the place-of-production change. Notice that /z/ → [s] changed only voicing; place and manner remained the same. The change from [s] → [t] provided the manner change from a fricative to a stop; voice and place of production were the same. Then the change from [t] → [ʔ] represented the change in place of production; voice and manner were the same. Each process only changed one aspect of consonant production: place, voice, or manner. All three phonological processes were required to account for Cameron's error in production to account for the fact that all three parameters of consonant production were altered.

Edwards (1992) describes the occurrence of multiple processes affecting a single sound change as "process density." The further removed a child's production is from the adult target, the more phonological processes there are affecting that production. Edwards discusses a metric that accounts for the number of processes applied within a given word as well as within a single sound change. This metric is called *process density index* (PDI), and it provides a rough measure of phonological severity. This measure represents the average number of phonological processes that are used per word. It is calculated by adding the total number of phonological processes that occur for all words in the sample and dividing by the total number of words. Using our two previous examples as a minisample, there were a total of six phonological processes (2 + 4) that occurred on our sample of two words. The PDI would be 3 (6 ÷ 2 = 3). The PDI can be used with any speech sample to provide a rough measure of phonological severity. Obviously, the higher the PDI, the more severe the speech disorder. One caution is needed, however. Because PDI does not account for qualitative differences across phonological processes, all processes are given equal value, or weight.

Thus, a common substitution process, such as t/s, would be given the same value for severity as a more idiosyncratic process, such as w/s. The more unusual process, however, would affect intelligibility—and therefore severity—to a greater extent than the more common substitution. This same problem is also present in omission errors and substitution errors. An omission error affects intelligibility and represents a more severe disorder than a substitution error, but both are weighted equally according to the PDI. In fact, a child with substitution errors could have a higher PDI if more processes are required to account for his or her sound error. With these limitations in mind, the PDI can be used as a rough measure of phonological severity.

The final step in the phonological process analysis is to organize and summarize the results of the analysis. A summary sheet, similar to one described by Elbert and Gierut (1986), organizes the processes according to syllable structure processes (deletion), sound simplification processes (substitution and assimilation), and other processes (idiosyncratic). The results of the analysis are summarized by totaling the number of occurrences of each process on the sheet. Also included on the sheet are the relative ages at which the processes are suppressed according to Grunwell (1987).

Edwards (1994) suggests that additional information also be provided that describes more specifically how the processes are applied in a particular speech sample for a given child. This should include information regarding process limitation or application, with regard to the class or classes of sounds affected by a process and the position(s) in which the process is applied. In addition, information should be provided regarding the frequency of occurrence of a process. Frequency of occurrence is determined by reporting the number of times a process occurred out of the number of times that the process could have potentially occurred in the sample. Finally, Edwards suggests that developmental information be provided on the age appropriateness of a phonological process. Specifically, it should be noted if a process persists beyond the age at which it should have been suppressed. Space is allotted at the end of the phonological process summary sheet to provide this additional information.

The following summarizes the steps in completing a nonstandardized phonological process analysis:

1. Complete whole-word transcriptions on a speech sample.
2. Transcribe the target word according to the adult model.
3. Apply appropriate phonological processes in a sequential manner until all aspects of sound change are accounted.
4. Summarize the results on a summary sheet indicating the frequency of occurrence of each phonological process.
5. Select appropriate treatment target(s).

The results of Cameron's phonological process analysis are presented in Appendix 2.A. The results of this analysis are organized on the summary sheet in Appendix 2.B. Examining the summary sheet, it can be seen that Cameron used deletion, substitution, assimilation, and idiosyncratic processes. The most frequently occurring processes were cluster reduction, fronting, and glottal replacement.

Based on this analysis, what phonological processes should be targeted for intervention? There are different perspectives about choosing the most appropriate processes to target. One perspective is to select the most frequently occurring processes because these would have the greatest impact on intelligibility. Another option is to use a developmental perspective and select processes that have persisted beyond the age at which they should have been suppressed. A third option is to use a combination of these two perspectives and select developmentally appropriate processes that are also frequently occurring.

Two different phonological processes could be selected on the basis of frequency of occurrence and developmental level: fronting and glottal replacement. Specific targets affected by each of processes could include

Fronting:	d ~ g	word-initially
	s ~ ʃ	word-initially
Glottal replacement:	ʔ ~ p	word-finally
	ʔ ~ t	word-finally

A third possibility may include cluster reduction. An early cluster could be selected, such as [st]:

| Cluster reduction: | t ~ st | word-initially |

What are the advantages of a phonological process analysis? The greatest advantage of this analysis is that it provides a description of the error patterns that are present in a child's speech. This is a tremendous step forward from the previous sound-by-sound traditional analysis that would have simply listed each sound error independently of any relationship to other sounds. As a consequence, intervention is more efficient because treatment is directed to patterns affecting entire classes of sounds rather than to individual sounds.

One disadvantage of the phonological process analysis is the amount of time it requires to complete. Although the clinician becomes more proficient with experience, the results from this analysis are very similar to a less time-consuming analysis, the PVM analysis. Further, the selection of treatment targets from the summary sheet is not always so obvious or easy. A simple summary of the frequency of occurrence of processes often requires the clinician to refer back to the analysis to determine the specific application of a phonological process. Completing the additional summary suggested by Edwards (1994) alleviates some of this difficulty. However, it adds more time to completing each analysis.

Place-Voice-Manner Analysis
The PVM analysis provides a description of a child's patterns of error productions on the basis of three broad categories of consonant production: place, voice, and manner of articulation. This analysis was first described by Weber (1970) and later by Turton (1973). Clinicians may also be familiar

with this analysis, which is used in the commercial Fisher-Logemann Test of Articulation (Fisher & Logemann, 1971) and the Compton-Hutton Phonological Assessment (Compton & Hutton, 1978).

The PVM analysis is completed by transferring the data from the whole-word transcriptions to a PVM form (shown in Appendix 2.C). This form, developed by Thomas Powell at Indiana University in 1982, organizes the consonants according to manner (nasals, stops, fricatives, affricates, liquids, and glides) along the top of the form. Voicing is indicated by shading of the voiced consonants. Within each manner class, the consonants are listed according to place of production, from the most anterior to the most posterior.

Under each consonant there are three columns that correspond to the three syllable positions: prevocalic, intervocalic, and postvocalic. These syllable positions are labeled on the left margin of the form beside each column. Terms for syllable positions were used rather than the word positions of initial, medial, and final. For multisyllabic words such as *Christmas* and *bathtub*, syllable positions are better suited for describing arresting and releasing consonants rather than the more ambiguous label of *medial*. Shaded boxes represent syllable positions in which a particular consonant cannot occur in English. For example, [ŋ] cannot occur prevocalically, and [w,j,h] cannot occur postvocalically.

The bottom of the form contains boxes where target clusters can be examineC. The clusters are divided into nasal clusters, [l] clusters, [r] clusters, [w] clusters, and [s] clusters. Examples of specific clusters are listed at the bottom of each cluster box.

The final two boxes at the bottom right of the form provide spaces for the child's phonetic inventory and a summary of the predominant error patterns according to place, voice, and manner categories.

Before completing the PVM analysis exercise, a couple of final comments are worth noting. First, the PVM analysis is an assessment of consonant production, with the exception of vocalic [l, r]. Occurrences of vocalic [l], stressed and unstressed [ɝ, ɚ], and the family of diphthong [r]s can be recorded in the boxes for consonantal [l] and [r].

The final note is to use color coding to increase the visualization of error patterns identified by this analysis. Tally marks in black or blue ink can be used for correct productions, and a red pen can be used to write in the child's error productions. At the completion of the analysis, a visible pattern of the child's errors can be more easily identified.

To begin this analysis, first code Cameron's consonant productions from the whole-word transcriptions on the Goldman-Fristoe Test of Articulation to the PVM analysis form. Using blue or black for correct productions and red for errored productions, you are ready to begin. Proceed word by word and within each word, consonant by consonant, until you have completed all of the child's responses. Moving from left to right, mark each consonant with the appropriate color in the appropriate box. For the first item, "house," use the blue pen to place a tally mark in the prevocalic box under the phoneme [h]; also place a blue tally mark in the postvocalic box under the phoneme [s]. This indicates correct production of both the prevocalic and postvocalic consonants in this word. Let's try a word that has some errored productions. In the second item, "telephone," write [d] in red under the prevocalic [t] box; write "φ" in the [l] intervocalic box to indicate omission; and make blue tally marks for intervocalic [f] and postvocalic [n] to indicate correct production of these two sounds. Proceed through the list of words in the same manner. Remember to mark clusters in the appropriate boxes.

After you have completed the list of words, use the phonetic inventory box to write the sounds produced by the child. It is recommended that you use the criterion specified by Stoel-Gammon (1987) and others that a sound must occur at least two times to be included in the phonetic inventory. Sounds that occur fewer than two times can be listed in the inventory as marginal sounds. This can be indicated by placing the marginal sounds in parentheses. It is also recommended that you include sounds produced by the child regardless of their accuracy relative to the adult target. In other words, the phonetic inventory is a listing of sounds produced by the child independent of his or her accuracy to the adult target.

In the final box, write the predominant error patterns that were noted according to errors of place, voice, or manner. When you have completed the analysis, compare your results with the answer sheet in Appendix 2.C.

What patterns were evident in Cameron's sound system according to this analysis? Visual inspection of the PVM form reveals that Cameron had particular difficulty with *manner* of consonant production, specifically fricatives, affricates, and occasionally liquids. With regard to *place* of production, Cameron had difficulty with posterior obstruents, namely palatals and velars. *Voicing* errors were limited primarily to intervocalic position in which he frequently produced the voiceless glottal stop [ʔ] for all consonants, voiced and voiceless.

Other error patterns can be detected on this form as well. Notice the cluster errors listed in each cluster category at the bottom of the form. Only one cluster, [tr], was produced correctly. All other clusters were reduced or occasionally simplified. A second pattern can be seen on this form that involves the omission or glottalization of postvocalic consonants.

These error patterns can be visualized from the PVM form and summarized according to the three broad categories of consonant production:

Place: Palatals and velars are replaced with alveolars.
Voice: Voiced and voiceless consonants are replaced with the voiceless glottal stop intervocalically.
Manner: Affricates and the voiceless velar stop are replaced by fricatives word-initially.
Other: Clusters are replaced by singletons.
         Final consonants are omitted or glottalized.

Finally, the phonetic inventory is completed to specify Cameron's sound inventory. Notice that his phonetic inventory is relatively complete with the exception of posterior obstruents [k, g, ʃ, tʃ, dʒ].

Based on the PVM analysis, what targets would be selected for intervention? The place and manner errors can both be addressed in one goal by selecting [k] word-initially. Another goal might be to address the omission of final consonants, such as [d]. However, addressing a voiced stop word-finally frequently results in the addition of schwa [ʌ] word-finally (e.g., [dɑgʌ]). Another option might be to address cluster production. An early cluster to start with would be [st]. These goals are summarized thus:

Goal 1:   s ~ k   word-initially
Goal 2:   t ~ st   word-initially

Advantages of the PVM analysis include that it is relatively simple and quick to complete. The visual representation of the analysis, however, is its most functional advantage. Patterns are easily identified by the color coding of errors and the organization of the form according to place, manner, and voicing of English consonants. Selection of targets for intervention is enhanced by the visual display of the completed analysis. This form also provides a useful tool for communicating results to parents or other professionals. Finally, the form is useful in comparing pre- and postintervention phonological analyses.

A disadvantage of the PVM analysis is that it does not identify assimilation errors, whereas the phonological process analysis does. The PVM analysis also does not provide a description of syllable structure or deletion processes, although these patterns can be identified on the PVM analysis form. For example, deletion of final consonants would be noted by red null (φ) indicators in the postvocalic row on the PVM form.

The following is a summary of the steps involved in completing a PVM analysis:

1.   Complete whole-word transcriptions on a speech sample.
2.   Use black and red markers to color code the analysis.
3.   Moving from left to right, mark each consonant with the appropriate color in the appropriate box. Correct consonant productions are tallied with the black marker; the red marker is used to write the incorrect productions.
4.   List the child's phonetic inventory using Stoel-Gammon's (1987) criterion of two occurrences per sound to be included in the inventory.
5.   Summarize the error patterns according to place, voice, and manner of consonant production.
6.   Select appropriate treatment target(s).

Comparison of the Relational Analyses
The phonological process analysis and the PVM analysis provided similar descriptions of Cameron's speech. The PVM error patterns can easily be renamed using phonological process terms. A summary comparison of the two analyses can be found in Table 2.3.

Notice that both analyses described the same error patterns. Only the terms used to describe the patterns were different. The phonological processes were easier, more descriptive terms; hence, the greater acceptance and use of phonological processes.

The differences between the two analyses included the lack of a phonological process to describe the replacement of the voiceless velar

TABLE 2.3 Summary comparison of the phonological process analysis and the place-voice-manner analysis of Cameron's speech

Place-voice-manner error patterns	Phonological processes
Palatals and velars are replaced by alveolars	Fronting
Affricates and voiceless velar stops are replaced by fricatives	Deaffrication; idiosyncratic
Liquids are replaced by glides	Gliding
Intervocalic consonants are replaced by glottal stops	Glottal replacement; idiosyncratic
Clusters are replaced by singletons	Cluster reduction
Consonants are omitted or glottalized word-finally	Final consonant deletion; glottal replacement

stop by [s] and replacement of intervocalic consonants with [ʔ]. The process analysis was limited to describing both of these error patterns as "idiosyncratic."

The summary sheet for the phonological process analysis was separate from the actual analysis. This separation made it more difficult to select treatment targets. Additionally, fronting encompassed several types of errors—for example, fronting of velars, fronting of palatals, and fronting of alveolars. To select a specific target from this process, the clinician must go back to the original data to determine which sounds were fronted and then decide on the target. This separation of the summary from the analysis was further accentuated in the label of *cluster reduction*. Frequently, cluster reduction refers to the deletion of one consonant from the cluster, e.g., [tɑp] for "stop." For Cameron, cluster reduction frequently involved the reduction of the cluster to a third consonant that was neither of the target consonants (e.g., [fʌθ] for "brush"). As noted previously, the PVM analysis and the summary were the same, whereas the process analysis required several pages to complete and was separate from the summary sheet.

In addition to the occasional differences in terminology and the summary differences, there is a final comparison between the two analyses. How much time did it take to complete each analysis? The PVM analysis took much less time than the process analysis and yielded similar results. The reason the PVM analysis took less time is because no labeling was required for any of the sound errors. The simple tallying/coding of consonant productions required much less time than the labeling of each sound change using a list of phonological processes.

Independent Analysis + Relational Analysis

As noted previously, an independent analysis examines a child's sound system as a unique, self-contained system without reference to the adult system. Independent analyses for describing the speech of late talkers have been discussed by Stoel-Gammon (1994). This type of analysis has been used with late talkers largely because of the variability of their immature sound systems, which results in a lack of a stable one-to-one correspondence between their sound productions and the adult targets. In early phonological acquisition, children are learning a sound system primarily by using a whole-word strategy rather than by a segmental rule-based approach. The independent analysis provides information on the sounds produced by the child (i.e., phonetic inventory) and the syllable structures produced by the child.

Independent analyses have been incorporated in the description of disordered sound systems (Williams, 1993). The independent analysis indicates the permissible sounds and sound sequences in a child's own sound system. In this regard, the independent analysis examines a child's sound system as a unique, "exotic," self-contained sound system.

The combination of an independent and relational analysis provides a more complete description of a child's speech. The relational analysis alone only provides a partial description—namely, what the child *cannot* do or what the child does incorrectly relative to the adult target. The independent analysis provides the other half of the picture—that is, what the child *can* do. The independent analysis is particularly useful to complete on children who have limited speech intelligibility.

It is important to complete an independent analysis as a first step in describing a child's speech. We can more fully understand a child's speech if we first have a description of the structure and organization of that system. Knowing this information provides us with a basis for then relating the child's system to the adult system in the relational analysis. By understanding the child's system first, we are able to discover the "order in the disorder" when comparing the two sound systems. As we will see in the next example, the mapping of the two sound systems (child to adult) provides a description as well as an explanation of the strategies developed by the child to compensate for a limited sound system. Although the child has developed her "own" language, it is the English language in which the child must communicate. How does she stretch a limited sound inventory to cover all the English consonants? The answers to these questions are available to us only when we can map the child's system onto the adult's system. The amazing, exciting, and challenging aspects of a speech analysis is the fact that each child develops a unique and creative strategy to accommodate his or her limited sound system. It is the goal of the speech-language pathologist to identify these compensatory strategies. Furthermore, it is the ultimate challenge of the speech-language pathologist to design an intervention plan that will use this information in helping the child restructure his or her sound system so that it matches the ambient or adult sound system.

There are different analyses that use independent + relational analyses in the assessment of children's speech. One approach that has been commonly reported in the literature is the assessment of productive phonological knowledge (Gierut et al., 1987; Gierut, 1986). This approach assesses productive phonological knowledge using the tenets of standard generative phonology to infer the nature of a child's underlying representations (or competence) from the child's productions (i.e., performance) on an extensive list of words plus conversational sample.

Systemic analysis is another approach that also incorporates independent + relational analyses. This approach was described by Williams (1993) and incorporates aspects of Grunwell's (1987) work of mapping the child's system to the adult system. The systemic analysis makes no inferences about a child's knowledge of the ambient sound system. Rather, it attempts to describe the structure and organization of the child's sound system as it relates to the target or adult sound system. In other words, it describes the order in the disorder (Grunwell, 1997). The mapping of the child-to-adult sound systems further provides an initial explanatory account in terms of compensatory strategies developed by the child to communicate in the English language with their own "language" or limited sound system.

There are five components in completing a systemic analysis:

1. Phonetic inventory
2. Distribution of sounds
3. Identification of patterns relative to target cluster production
4. Mapping of the child-to-adult sound systems
5. Identifying organizational principles or strategies

I offer a helpful hint to make your analysis more efficient and easier to interpret: If you get in the habit of organizing your analyses (phonetic inventory, distribution, and mapping) according to place and manner of consonant production, then you will be able to identify gaps in the child's inventory and patterns in his or her organization much more easily. Specifically, organize sounds first according to manner of consonant production (i.e., stops, fricatives, etc.). Then organize sounds according to place of production within each manner classification, going from the most anterior to the most posterior place of production (i.e., labial, alveolar, velar for the stops). Remember, the goal of an analysis is to identify patterns in the child's sound system. The more organized your analysis, the better you will be able to identify the patterns in the child's speech.

The first step in the systemic analysis is to list the child's phonetic inventory *independently* of the accuracy of his or her productions. To provide additional information, it is useful to construct separate phonetic inventories for word-initial and word-final positions. Stoel-Gammon (1987) recommends using a criterion of a minimum of two occurrences of each sound in each word position for a sound to be included in the phonetic inventory.

The second step in the systemic analysis is to examine the distribution of sounds in the child's language. Although the child may not produce all the English sounds (as noted in the phonetic inventory you have just completed), list all English sounds and indicate what the child does for each sound/position. This provides the basis for your mapping. The distribution form is the bottom part of the form used for the phonetic inventory, as shown in the completed analysis in Appendix 2.D. Notice that the sounds are listed along the left side according to manner and then place within each manner category. Along the top of the distribution form are linguistic notations to indicate word or syllable position. The following notations indicate the position of the target sound within word positions or syllable positions:

- Word-initial (prevocalic) # ____
- Word-medial (intervocalic) V ____ V
- Word-final (postvocalic) ____ #

On this form, indicate the presence, absence, or marginal occurrence of a particular sound in a given syllable or word position. Use the following notation to specify this information for each sound in each position:

1. The presence of a sound in a given position is indicated by an X.
2. The absence of a sound in a given position is indicated by an open box "❑."
3. The marginal occurrence of a sound in a given position is indicated by a fraction that specifies how many times the sound was produced out of the total number of times the sound occurred in the sample. Example: "5/7" indicates that the child correctly produced the target sound in that position five times out of seven opportunities.

For the absence or marginal occurrence of a target sound in a given position (2 and 3), indicate what sound(s) the child produced. Write above the box or fraction the sound produced by the child. This provides the basis for the mapping that we will do in the fourth step.

The third step is to identify patterns in the child's production of target clusters. At the end of the distribution form is a section to note this. To be able to identify patterns in the child's production of clusters, it is necessary to organize target clusters according to type. For example, stop and fricative clusters can be classified into categories (Table 2.4).

Children develop different strategies in compensating for target cluster production just as they do for a limited phonetic inventory and distribution of English consonants. They may develop rules that correspond to specific target clusters, such as "stop + liquid" and "fricative + liquid." However, they may also develop rules that are broader than these categories and encompass all "consonant + sonorant" clusters, which would include all the clusters in Table 2.4 except "fricative + stop" clusters. Some children, as we will see with Cameron, may be somewhere between these two extremes and be a little more specific on the first consonant, but not

TABLE 2.4   Stop and fricative clusters categories

Stop clusters	Fricative clusters	Broad classification
Stop + liquid	Fricative + liquid	
Stop + glide	Fricative + glide	C + sonorant
	Fricative + nasal	
	Fricative + stop	C + obstruent

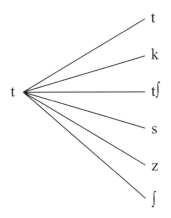

FIGURE 2.1   *Example of a 1:6 phoneme collapse.*

on the second consonant of the target cluster. For example, a child may have a rule that differentiates the first consonant of the cluster on the basis of place and manner of production. "Labial stops + sonorants are produced as [f]" would be an example of a rule that provides a more specific classification of the first "C," but the second "C," sonorants, remains unspecified.

With practice you will become more proficient in identifying cluster patterns. You may simply list what the child is doing for each target cluster category initially and then review the list to identify any similarities across categories that then could be written as a broader rule.

The fourth step is to map the child's system onto the adult's system by diagramming phoneme collapses. Typical speakers have a one-to-one correspondence between a target sound and their production. Children who have a speech disorder frequently collapse several adult phonemic contrasts into a single sound in their sound system. This results in a one-to-many correspondence. For example, a child may produce [t] for several adult sounds, including [t, k, tʃ, s, z, ʃ]. In this case, the child has collapsed six different adult sounds into one sound: [t]. This phonemic collapse can be diagrammed, as shown in Figure 2.1.

To determine the phoneme collapses that are present in a child's system, return to the distribution of sounds that you completed. A form for diagramming the phoneme collapses is included in Part III of Appendix 2.D. Notice that the phoneme collapses are diagrammed by position. Look down the word-initial, or prevocalic, column on your distribution form. Do you see a sound that was used frequently for other target sounds in that position? Weiner (1982) referred to this as a sound preference. If you see one, write the sound produced by the child on your phoneme collapse form under the word-initial, or prevocalic, position. Then diagram all the target sounds that were produced by the child with that one sound. Remember to list these sounds in an organized fashion, all in one manner category and according to place within the manner category. If the child used the sound target appropriately, list that sound first. Con-

FIGURE 2.2   *Phoneme collapses of target voiceless and voiced continuants.*

tinue diagramming the phoneme collapses through all word or syllable positions. Target clusters would be included in the collapses if the child produced the cluster with the same sound preference as you are diagramming the target singleton collapses.

The final step in the systemic analysis is to identify organizational principles that are present in the child's structure of his or her phonological system. Generally, children organize their systems relative to the adult sound system with regard to place, manner, and voicing. One or more of these characteristics can be the basis of a child's organizational scheme. An example may help to demonstrate this concept. A child, Mark, age 6;0 (example taken from Grunwell, 1987) exhibited a sound preference for [h] word-initially for voiceless fricatives. For voiced continuants (fricatives and liquids), he produced [j]. These phoneme collapses are diagrammed in Figure 2.2.

In this example, notice that Mark retained two aspects of the ambient production in his system: voicing and, broadly, manner. Specifically, voiceless continuants (i.e., voiceless fricatives) were collapsed to a voiceless continuant, [h]. Voiced continuants (i.e., liquids) were collapsed to a voiced continuant, [j]. This is remarkable! The child attended to these two aspects (i.e., voicing and manner) from the ambient sound system and constructed a compensatory strategy to accommodate those sounds that were absent from his limited sound system. Even more remarkable is the symmetry that Mark maintained. Voiceless continuants were produced with a voiceless continuant; voiced continuants were produced with a voiced continuant. The "logic" in Mark's structure is incredibly amazing! As you can see, this is the truly amazing and challenging aspect of describing and *explaining* the child's system. It *is* systematic, structured, ordered, organized, and predictable.

In sum, we can describe the organizational principles for this sample of Mark's speech as voicing and manner. Specifically, voiceless continuants were collapsed to the voiceless continuant, [h]; voiced continuants were collapsed to the voiced continuant, [j].

It should be noted that this was a limited sample of only 20 words that Grunwell selected to illustrate a particular aspect of Mark's speech. Consequently, several target sounds were not included in this brief sample. One could hypothesize, however, that based on this pattern, Mark would produce voiced fricatives [ð, z] as [j] because they are also voiced continuants. Because there are no voiceless continuants that are not fricatives, no additional sounds can be added to the [h] collapse unless it was the voiceless fricative, [θ].

Let's summarize the steps involved in completing a systemic phonological analysis. These include

1. Construct an independent phonetic inventory for each position (word-initial, word-medial, word-final). Use phonetic inventory form (see Part I; Appendix 2.D).
2. List the distribution of the child's sounds relative to the ambient system. Use distribution form (see Part II; Appendix 2.D).
   a. Indicate, by position, the presence, absence, or marginal occurrence of each target sound.
   b. For sounds that are absent or marginal, indicate what sound the child produces for that target sound and position.
3. Specify the child's production of target clusters. Use cluster form (see Part II; Appendix 2.D).
   a. Identify patterns of target cluster productions.
   b. Describe patterns of target cluster productions using specific or broad classification.
4. Map the child's system to the adult system. Use phoneme collapse form (see Part III; Appendix 2.D).
   a. Look for sound preferences by position on the distribution form.
   b. Diagram phoneme collapses by position.
   c. Include target clusters in phoneme collapses, if appropriate.
5. Identify organizational principles operating in child's system.
   a. Examine phoneme collapses to identify compensatory strategies developed by the child that generally correspond to place, voice, and manner of the ambient system.
   b. Look for ordered, organized, predictable, logical, and symmetrical patterns.
6. Select targets for intervention.

After you have completed a systemic phonological analysis on Cameron's speech sample, compare your results to the key in Appendix 2.D. What patterns were evident? What organizational principles were identified for the structure of Cameron's sound system?

Cameron's phonetic inventory was fairly well represented by all classes, with the exception of affricates. With regard to place of production, posterior consonants, such as palatal fricative, affricates, and velar stops, were missing. Word-initial and word-final inventories were relatively equivalent. Cameron had several marginal sounds in his inventory; however, this may be an artifact of the test, which did not have more than a single exemplar for each target sound per position.

Visual inspection of the sound distribution indicates that Cameron was missing several sounds. Although Cameron produced some of these sounds as indicated in the phonetic inventory, he may not have produced them target appropriately or produced them in all target positions. Closer examination of the distribution reveals a pattern within a particular class of sounds. Specifically, Cameron had more difficulty with word-initial voiceless stops than voiced stops. Notice that he produced the anterior voiceless stops with voicing, whereas anterior voiced stops were produced correctly. Another pattern is observed word-finally with voiced and voiceless stops. Voiceless stops were produced as a glottal stop, whereas voiced stops were deleted. Velar stops were never produced in any position.

The distribution of Cameron's sound productions reveals that he had more difficulty with sounds postvocalically (i.e., medial and final word positions). The majority of target intervocalic consonants was produced as a glottal stop, and final consonants were frequently omitted.

Cameron's cluster production is summarized at the bottom of the form. His production of target clusters can be captured basically by three complementary rules. These rules are

1. C_{labial} + son → [f]
   (labial consonants + sonorant clusters are typically produced as [f])
2. $C_{nonlabial}$ + son → [s]
   (nonlabial consonants + sonorant clusters are typically produced as [s])
3. [s] + C → [s]
   ([s] + consonant clusters are typically produced as [s])

These rules appear to be motivated by phonetic assimilation in that the nature of the first ambient consonant as labial or nonlabial typically influenced Cameron's production as a labial, [f], or nonlabial, [s].

Mapping of Cameron's sound system to the adult system revealed extensive phoneme collapses, as shown on Part III of Appendix 2.D. Diagramming the phoneme collapses according to place within manner of consonant production reveals the systematic and logical nature of Cameron's sound system. Specifically, primarily voiced obstruents were collapsed to [d] word-initially, whereas voiceless obstruents were collapsed to [s]. Notice that Cameron maintained the characteristics of the ambient sounds that were collapsed—that is, voiced obstruents were collapsed to a voiced obstruent (i.e., [d]), and voiceless obstruents were collapsed to a voiceless obstruent (i.e., [s]). The third extensive collapse word-initially involved the collapse of primarily labial consonant + sonorant clusters to a labial, [f].

Intervocalically, Cameron collapsed voiced and voiceless consonants (sonorants and obstruents) to glottal stop. Notice that he had less specificity in this position than in word-initial or word-final positions. This tends to indicate that Cameron's sound system was less developed intervocalically than in the more salient initial and final word positions. Neither voicing nor type of consonant was specified by this collapse.

Word-finally, Cameron again collapsed ambient sounds with regard to their nature and voicing characteristics. Similar to his word-initial collapses, primarily voiced obstruents were collapsed, but in this position, they were collapsed to null. Voiceless obstruents were collapsed to glottal stops.

Based on these phoneme collapses, the following principles may be identified as possible organizational schemes or strategies to accommodate Cameron's limited sound system:

1. Voicing of obstruents by position, with the exception of intervocalic position
   a. Word-initial
      (1) $V^{-}_{obs} \rightarrow [s] / \#$ ___
          Voiceless obstruents are collapsed to [s] word-initially.
      (2) $V^{+}_{obs} \rightarrow [d] / \#$ ___
          Voiced obstruents are collapsed to [d] word-initially.
   b. Word-medial
      (1) $C \rightarrow ? / V$ ___ V
          Consonants are collapsed to glottal stop word-medially.
   c. Word-final
      (1) $V^{-}_{obs} \rightarrow ?$ ___ $\#$
          Voiceless obstruents are collapsed to glottal stop word-finally.
      (2) $V^{+}_{obs} \rightarrow \phi /$ ___ $\#$
          Voiced obstruents are collapsed to null word-finally.
2. Production of clusters as singletons
   a. $C_{labial} + son \rightarrow [f]$
      Labial consonants + sonorant clusters are produced as [f].
   b. $C_{nonlabial} + sonorant \rightarrow [s]$
      Nonlabial consonants + sonorant clusters are produced as [s].
   c. $[s] + C \rightarrow [s]$
      [s] + consonant clusters are produced as [s].

Given the systemic analysis, we have more knowledge about Cameron's sound system from a descriptive perspective than we gained from either of the two relational analyses. We also have some possible explanatory accounts for the organization of his sound system that were not available from either of the two previous analyses. With this analysis, we are able to see how Cameron's system relates to the adult system through the mapping of the two systems. Notice that this analysis is child based rather than adult based. No *a priori* labels or categories were required to describe Cameron's sound system in relation to the ambient system. This allows the clinician to view the child's system more holistically as the *child* has organized his or her own system. The collapses noted in mapping Cameron's system to the adult system would have been fragmented by the phonological process labels or broad categories of place, voice, and manner of the previous analyses. For example, the collapse of voiceless obstruents to [s] word-initially would have had *six* different phonological processes to account for all the sound changes included in this *one* collapse. These include

1. Devoicing (s/z)
2. Fronting (s/ʃ)
3. Idiosyncratic (s/k)
4. Deaffrication + fronting (s/tʃ)
5. Cluster reduction (s/sk; s/st)
6. Cluster reduction + idiosyncratic (s/kl)

Six different phonological processes were needed to describe *one* pattern in the child's system. These processes miss the fact that all the sound changes were related to a single pattern. Further, they miss the organizational principle on which these sounds were collapsed—specifically, that voiceless obstruents were collapsed to a voiceless obstruent and how this collapse complements the other collapses in Cameron's system to form a logical and organized system. Finally, selection of appropriate treatment targets is influenced by the different analyses. As discussed previously, phonological processes are selected on the basis of frequency of occurrence and by developmental norms. This may not take into account the child's organization of his or her own system and bases target selection on data that are more removed from what the child actually does. We must first understand the *organization* of a child's system to effectively *reorganize* it through intervention.

Based on the systemic analysis, what targets would be selected for intervention? Some guidelines have been developed for selection of appropriate treatment targets (Williams, 1998) that have the potential of maximum reorganization and thus result in increases in intelligibility. These include

- Select idiosyncratic collapses.
- Select sounds from extensive phoneme collapses.
- Select sounds that are most representative of the phoneme collapse error pattern.
- Select sounds that are *maximally distinct* from the child's production in terms of place, voice, and manner.
- Select sounds using *maximal classification*—that is, sounds that are from different sound classes (*manner*), different *places* of production, and different *voicing*.
- Select sounds that result in meaningful sound contrasts.

Using these guidelines, the following targets could be selected for intervention:

$$k \sim s \mathbin{/} \# \_\_\_$$
$$br \sim f \mathbin{/} \# \_\_\_$$
$$z \sim ? \mathbin{/} V \_\_\_ V$$

Notice that these targets address two word positions, singletons and consonant clusters, stops and fricatives, and voiced and voiceless sounds. Also notice how diverse (maximally different) the target is from the comparison sound. In the first goal, [k] is different from [s] in terms of place and manner; in the second goal, [br] is different from [f] in terms of place, voice, manner, and singleton versus cluster; and in the third goal, [z] is different from [?] in terms of place, voice, and manner. By addressing idiosyncratic and extensive phoneme collapses, intervention has the potential of having a major impact on the child's phonological structure or organization. Further, selection of specific sound targets on the basis of maximal distinction and maximal classification make the target sounds more salient and thereby potentially more learnable.

Notice that developmental norms were not included in the guidelines for target selection. In a study by Gierut et al. (1996), it was suggested that selection of treatment sounds on the basis of developmental factors incorporates subordinate properties of the sound system and therefore does not induce sound change to the extent of superordinate properties, such as implicational, dynamic, or cognitive factors.

*Sub*ordinate properties would include factors such as age of acquisition and ease of production. *Super*ordinate properties, on the other hand, consider factors such as markedness and implicational rules, linguistic principles that govern all human languages, the hierarchal structure of phonetic features within a sound system, and the learnability of new contrasts based on the existing phonological structure. The guidelines listed previously take superordinate factors into account in structuring intervention to result in the greatest amount of reorganization of the child's sound system.

What are the advantages of a systemic analysis? This analysis provides a detailed description of sound systems that are severe to profoundly impaired as a result of extensive gaps in a child's sound system relative to the ambient system. It is a *child-based* analysis rather than an *adult-based* analysis. Thus, the numerous sound errors do not need to be labeled or categorized according to a finite set of *a priori* adult-based labels. It can therefore describe idiosyncratic errors not captured by common phonological processes. Consequently, the systemic analysis also provides a holistic assessment of the child's speech because the child's patterns are not fragmented into the *a priori* set of labels. The systemic analysis provides descriptive and explanatory accounts of the child's system through examination of organizational principles that reflect unique strategies developed by the child to compensate for a restricted sound system.

Comparison of Analyses

It was noted previously that the two relational analyses—phonological process analysis and PVM analysis—yielded similar results despite different terminology. The independent + relational analysis—systemic analysis—however, provided a much richer description of Cameron's sound system than either of the relational analyses. In addition, the systemic analysis provided an explanatory account of Cameron's sound system in terms of organizational principles that he developed to compensate for a system that was restricted relative to the ambient.

How do the analyses compare with each other in terms of selection of treatment targets? The treatment targets are summarized in Table 2.5 for each analysis for comparison.

Looking across the three analyses, you can see that two of them shared one common target for intervention. The process analysis and the PVM both selected t ~ st; and PVM and systemic analyses both selected s ~ k. Although no other shared targets occurred, there were shared error patterns selected for intervention. All three analyses selected the pattern of clusters, and the glottalization pattern was similar between the process and systemic analyses.

TABLE 2.5 Summary of treatment targets for three analyses

Phonological process	Place-voice-manner	Systemic
Fronting	Place + manner	Collapse of V̄ obstruents to [s]/#
d ~ g / # ___	s ~ k / # ___	s ~ k / # ___
s ~ ʃ / # ___		
Glottal replacement		Collapse of consonants to [ʔ]/V__V
ʔ ~ p / ___ #		ʔ ~ z / V__V
ʔ ~ t / ___ #		
Cluster reduction	Clusters	Collapse of labial stop+son to [f]/#__
t ~ st / # ___	t ~ st / # ___	f ~ br / # ___

Another way to compare the three analyses is in terms of ease of completion. Of the three, the PVM analysis required the least skill and use of terminology to complete the analysis. Recall that the analysis was completed by color coding the errors on an organized form. The coding was simple and quick and did not require labeling of the errored productions. The phonological process analysis took considerably more time to complete and provided similar results as the PVM analysis. The systemic analysis was similar to the PVM analysis with regard to relative ease in completing. Both analyses were essentially mechanisms for organizing the child's data to discover patterns. Neither required labeling, which is the greater time demand for analyzing speech patterns.

A final difference among the three analyses involves the amount of linguistic knowledge required to complete each analysis. The phonological process analysis and the systemic analysis both required some background in linguistics to complete the analyses, whereas the PVM analysis did not.

Should one analysis be chosen over the others, or are some analyses better suited for a particular population of children with speech disorders? Generally, the relational analyses provide adequate descriptions of children with mild to moderate speech disorders. Smaller speech samples are sufficient to analyze mild to moderate speech disorders, and the broad categories of PVM or the phonological processes are adequate to describe these sound systems and plan intervention programs. However, for children with numerous speech errors who have extensive gaps in their sound systems, a larger speech sample is needed to determine the patterns and principles on which their systems are organized. Additionally, an independent and relational analysis is required to first determine the organization of the child's system and to then contrast his or her organization to the adult system. Understanding the child's organization is essential in determining the most appropriate plan to reorganize his or her system and bringing it into a closer one-to-one correspondence with the adult or ambient sound system.

Reference Information

This section provides a brief review of reference information in the assessment of children's speech. Areas in which a speech-language pathologist may want to refer in completing an assessment include published test instruments, age norms for English consonants, and dialectal variations.

Published Test Instruments

The majority of the published tests used by speech-language pathologists to assess children's speech is based on an inventory of all English sounds occurring in all word positions. Many of these test instruments provide information regarding developmental norms on the age of acquisition of these sounds. Some tests were developed to assess error patterns. Still others are designed specifically to assess non-English speakers, primarily Spanish speakers. Finally, several tests have computerized versions for ease of scoring.

Several of these tests have been listed in Table 2.6 as a reference for speech-language pathologists. They are organized according to sound inventory tests, pattern tests, computerized tests, and non-English phonology tests. Most of the tests are summarized according to type of sample (words, sentences, conversation, etc.); sample size; ages of children for whom the test would be appropriate; recommended level of severity for which the test would be most appropriate; and type of analyses that could be completed on each test (e.g., relational or independent and then specific analysis). Information was not available for all of the published tests included in this table.

Age Norms for English Consonant Acquisition

A number of studies have been conducted to determine the age at which typically developing children acquire the consonants of the English language. These studies are generally cross-sectional, in which a large number of children at different age levels are tested at a single point in time on their ability to produce speech sounds. The investigators establish a criterion for determining "age of acquisition" for the group as a whole. Some studies use a stringent criterion level of 90% accuracy; others use a 75% criterion level; still others use a 50% criterion level to reflect "customary production" rather than "mastery" (Sander, 1972). The studies also differ in methodology used to collect the normative data, such as imitation versus spontaneous productions, reporting "full" versus "partial" data from children, and number of positions assessed (i.e., initial, medial, and final). Differences in criterion levels and methodology used to establish norms are very important to consider, because relatively small differences in methodology can greatly affect the age of acquisition reported by the studies. Further, studies of small groups of children have confirmed that individual differences across children are so great that it may be impossible to establish meaningful age norms. Therefore, it would be

TABLE 2.6 List of published test instruments

Tests	Type of sample	Sample size	Appropriate ages	Recommended severity level	Analyses
Sound inventory tests					
ALPHA (Assessment Link Between Phonology and Articulation) Phonology Test, Revised; Robert J. Lowe, 1995; ALPHA Speech and Language Resources	Delayed sentence imitation	50 target words embedded in short sentences	3–8 yrs	Mild to moderate	R:PPA
Fisher-Logemann Test of Articulation and Competence; Hilda Fisher and Jeri Logemann, 1971; Pro-Ed	Words/sentences	109 words, 15 sentences	3–80[+] yrs	Mild to moderate	R:DFA
Arizona Articulation Proficiency Scale, 2nd ed. (AAPS-2); Janet Fudala and William Reynolds, 1986; Western Psychological Services	Words	48 words, 25 sentences	1.6–13.11 yrs	Mild to moderate	R
Goldman-Fristoe Test of Articulation (GFTA); Ronald Goldman & Macalyne Fristoe, 1986; AGS	Words/sentences	35 words, 9 sentences	2–16[+] yrs	Mild to moderate	R:PPA/PVM
Photo Articulation Test, 2nd ed. (PAT-2); Kathleen Pendergast, Stanley Dickey, John Selmar, and Anton Soder, 1984; Pro-Ed	Words	72 words	3.6–8 yrs	Mild to moderate	R
Templin-Darley Test of Articulation; Mildred Templin and Fredic Darley, 1969; Speech Bin	Words/sentences	141 words	3–8 yrs	Mild to moderate	R
Test of Minimal Articulation Competence (T-MAC); Wayne Secord, 1981; Psychological Corporation	Words	107 items	3–80[+] yrs	Mild to moderate	R
Weiss Comprehensive Articulation Test (WCAT); Curtis Weiss, 1980; Pro-Ed	Words	50 words	Preschool–adult	Mild to moderate	R
Pattern tests					
Assessment of Phonological Processes-Revised (APP-R); Barbara Williams Hodson, 1986; Pro-Ed	Words	50 words	3–12 yrs	Moderate to severe	R:PPA
Bankson-Bernthal Test of Phonology (BBTOP); Nicholas Bankson and John Bernthal, 1990; Riverside Publishing Co.	Words	80 words	3.0–9.11 yrs	Mild to moderate	R:PPA
Khan-Lewis Phonological Analysis (KLPA); Linda Khan and Nancy Lewis, 1986; AGS	Words	44 words	2–5.11 yrs	Mild to moderate	R:PPA
Natural Process Analysis (NPA); Lawrence Shriberg and Joan Kwiatkowski, 1980; John Wiley	Spontaneous speech sample	100 different words (min.)	—	Mild to severe	R:PPA
Phonological Assessment of Child Speech (PACS); Pamela Grunwell, 1986; College-Hill Press	Spontaneous speech	100 words (min.); 200–250 words preferred	Preschool–school-age	Mild to severe	R:PPA

TABLE 2.6   continued

Tests	Type of sample	Sample size	Appropriate ages	Recommended severity level	Analyses
Phonological Process Analysis (PPA); Fredrick Weiner, 1979; Pro-Ed	Delayed imitation words	—	—	Mild to moderate	R:PPA
Smit-Hand Articulation and Phonology Evaluation (SHAPE); Ann Smit and Linda Hand, 1996; Western Psychological Services	Words	—	3–9 yrs	Moderate to severe	R + I
Computerized tests					
Computerised Assessment of Phonological Processes (CAPP); Barbara Williams Hodson, 1985; Interstate Printers and Publishers	Same as APP-R	—	—	—	—
Computerized Profiling; Steven Long & Marc Fey, 1994; Psychological Corporation	Words	—	—	Mild to moderate	R:PPA
Logical International Phonetic Programs (LIPP); K. Oller and R. Delgado, 1990; Intelligent Hearing Systems	—	—	—	—	—
Macintosh Interactive System for Phonological Analysis (ISPA); Julie Masterson and Frank Pagan, 1992; Psychological Corporation	Words	—	Any age	Mild to moderate	R:PPA
Programs to Examine Phonetic and Phonologic Evaluation Records (PEPPER); Lawrence Shriberg, 1986; Lawrence Erlbaum	Words	—	—	Mild to severe	R:PPA
Tests of non-English phonology					
Assessment of Phonological Process–Spanish (AAP-S); Barbara Williams Hodson, 1986; Los Amigos Association	Words	—	—	Mild to moderate	R:PPA
Austin Spanish Articulation Test (ASAT); Elizabeth Carrow, 1974; Teaching Resources Corporation	Words	—	—	Mild to moderate	R
Spanish Articulation Measures-Revised (SAM); Larry Mattes, 1994; Academic Communication Associates	Words	—	School age	Mild to moderate	R:PPA

DFA = distinctive feature analysis; I = independent analysis; PPA = phonological process analysis; PVM = place-voice-manner analysis; R= relational analysis.

TABLE 2.7 Normative acquisition data of English consonants according to three studies (50%, 75%, and 90% accuracy)

Consonant	Prather et al. (1975)		Sander (1972)		Smit et al. (1990)	
	50%	90%	50%	90%	50%	75%
n	<24	24	<24	36	<36	<36
m	<24	28	<24	36	<36	<36
p	<24	28	<24	36	<36	<36
h	<24	28	<24	36	<36	<90
t	<24	32	24	>48	<36	<36
k	24	32	24	44	<36	<36
f	<24	36	32	48	<36	42
w	<24	40	<24	40	<36	<36
ŋ	<24	36	24	>48	<36	<90
b	24	36	<24	48	<36	<36
g	24	36	24	48	<36	<36
s	24	44	36	>48	42	60
j	28	32	30	48	<36	42
d	28	36	24	48	<36	<36
hw	28	>48	Not assessed		Not assessed	
l	32	>48	36	>48	42	72
r	32	>48	36	>48	42	72
ʃ	36	>48	42	>48	42	60
tʃ	36	>48	42	>48	42	72
dʒ	36	>48	48	>48	42	54
v	40	>48	48	>48	42	54
z	44	>48	42	>48	48	72
ʒ	44	>48	44	>48	Not assessed	
ð	48	>48	48	>48	54	66
θ	48	>48	48	>48	54	72

Sources: Prather, E., Hedrick, D., & Kern, C. (1975). Articulation development in children aged two to four years. *Journal of Speech and Hearing Disorders, 40,* 179–191; Sander, E. (1972). When are speech sounds learned? *Journal of Speech and Hearing Disorders, 37,* 55–63; Smit, A., Hand, L., Frelinger, J., Bernthal, J., & Byrd, A. (1990). The Iowa articulation norms project and its Nebraska replication. *Journal of Speech and Hearing Disorders, 55,* 779–798.

a mistake to place a great deal of faith in an *exact age* at which a given sound can be expected to be produced correctly. Consequently, it is better to use norms as a *general* picture of acquisition.

With these caveats in mind, Table 2.7 summarizes the age norms across three different studies using three different criterion levels (50%, 75%, and 90%). Notice the similarities across studies, but also be aware of differences across both criterion levels and studies.

Dialectal Differences

To increase accuracy in assessment of children's speech, the speech-language pathologist must be aware of dialectal variations of Standard American English (SAE). Dialects are mutually intelligible forms of a language that are associated with a particular region, social class, or ethnic group. According to the American Speech-Language-Hearing Association's (1983) Position Paper on Social Dialects, there is no dialectal variety of English that is considered to be "a disorder or a pathological form of speech or language." It is, therefore, essential for speech-language pathologists to have information on the characteristics of particular languages and dialects, as well as information on normal phonological development, to provide nonbiased phonological assessments in differentiating children with *dialectal differences* from those with *phonological disorders.*

Examples of dialects spoken in the United States include

- African-American English
- Appalachian English
- Ozark English
- Mexican-American English
- Caribbean English

The characteristics of one dialect, African-American English, are summarized in Table 2.8.

Proctor (1994) discussed two diagnostic categories relative to cultural and phonological variation: (1) presence of a phonological difference (i.e., dialect) without a phonological disorder; and (2) presence of both a phonological difference and a phonological disorder. She defined a *phonological difference* as the speaker's first dialect (D_1) or first language (L_1) being different from SAE. Speakers with a phonological difference may shift (code mixing or code switching) from D_1 to D_2 or L_1 to L_2. Proctor summarizes that a *phonological disorder* is determined when one of three conditions is present:

1. The child's intelligibility is reduced to speakers within his or her speech community.
2. The child misarticulates sounds that are similar in both SAE and D_1 or L_1.
3. The child produces idiosyncratic patterns that are not characteristic of D_1, L_1, SAE, or of the code mixing or code switching processes.

Readers are encouraged to consult recent books and articles that cover this topic more comprehensively. Proctor (1994) provides a thorough and comprehensive discussion of cultural and linguistic variations in phonological assessment of children's speech.

TABLE 2.8 Characteristics of African-American vernacular English

Rule	Example (International Phonetic Alphabet)	Example (Orthography)
Word-final consonant cluster reduction	[tɛst] ~ [tɛs]	"test" ~ "tes"
Stopping of word-initial interdentals	[ðe] ~ [de]	"they" ~ "dey"
	[θɑt] ~ [tɑt]	"thought" ~ taught"
Substitution of f/θ and v/ð intervocalically	[nʌθɪŋ] ~ [nʌfiŋ]	"nothing" ~ "nofing"
	[beðɪŋ] ~ [beviŋ]	"bathing" ~ "baving"
Substitution of f/θ word-finally	[saʊθ] ~ [saʊf]	"south" ~ "souf"
Substitution of n/ŋ word-finally	[swɪŋ] ~ [swɪn]	"swing" ~ "swin"
Deletion of [r]	[sɪstɚ] ~ [sɪstə]	"sister" ~ "siste"
	[kærəl] ~ [kæəl]	"Carol" ~ "Caol"
	[prʌfɛsɚ] ~ [pʌfɛsə]	"professor" ~ pofesso"
Deletion of [l] in word-final clusters	[hɛlp] ~ [hɛp]	"help" ~ "hep"
Substitution of [ɪ] for [ɛ] before nasals	[pɛn] ~ [pɪn]	"pen" ~ "pin"
Deletion of nasals word-finally with nasalization of preceding vowel	[mun] ~ [mũ]	"moon" ~ "moo"
Devoicing of consonants word-finally	[bɛd] ~ [bɛt]	"bed" ~ "bet"

Source: Adapted from Iglesias, A., & Goldstein, B. (1998). Language and dialectal variations. In J. E. Bernthal & N. W. Bankson (Eds.), *Articulation and phonological disorders* (4th ed.) (148–171). Boston: Allyn & Bacon.

Conclusion

It is important for practitioners to use their clinical judgment in selecting analysis procedures that provide the best description for a given child. The speech pathologist must be aware of child factors that are important in selecting the most appropriate analysis procedure. Factors such as severity, age of child, and type of speech disability (articulation vs. phonological) are important considerations to take into account. Speech pathologists must learn different types of analyses and feel comfortable in using various approaches to improve their clinical practice. The material contained herein and the examples furnished in the book provide opportunities to learn some of the analysis approaches that are appropriate for different populations of children with speech disorders.

References

American Speech-Language-Hearing Association. (1983). Position of the American Speech-Language-Hearing Association on social dialects. *ASHA, 25,* 23–25.

Ball, M. J., & Kent, R. D. (1997). *The new phonologies: Developments in clinical linguistics.* San Diego: Singular Publishing Group, Inc.

Bernhardt, B., & Stoel-Gammon, C. (1994). Non-linear phonology: Introduction and clinical application: Tutorial. *Journal of Speech and Hearing Research, 37,* 123–143.

Bernthal, J., & Bankson, N. (1998). *Articulation and phonological disorders* (4th ed.). Englewood Cliffs, NJ: Prentice-Hall.

Compton, A. J., & Hutton, S. (1978). *Compton-Hutton phonological assessment.* San Francisco: Carousel House.

Dunn, C. (1982). Phonological process analysis: Contributions to assessing phonological disorders. *Communicative Disorders, 7,* 147–164.

Edwards, M. L. (1986, November). *Comprehensive procedures for phonological assessment.* Paper presented at the annual convention of the American Speech-Language-Hearing Association, Detroit, Michigan.

Edwards, M. L. (1992). In support of phonological processes: Clinical forum: Phonological assessment and treatment. *Language, Speech, and Hearing Services in Schools, 23,* 233–240.

Edwards, M. L. (1994). Phonological process analysis. In *Children's phonology disorders* (2nd ed.) (pp. 43–65). Rockville, MD: American Speech-Language-Hearing Association.

Elbert, M. (1992). Consideration of error types: A response to Fey. Clinical forum: Phonological assessment and treatment. *Language, Speech, and Hearing Services in Schools, 23,* 241–246.

Elbert, M., & Gierut, J. A. (1986). *Handbook of clinical phonology: Approaches to assessment and treatment.* San Diego: College Hill Press.

Fey, M. E. (1992). Articulation and phonology: Inextricable constructs in speech pathology. Clinical forum: Phonological assessment and treatment. *Language, Speech, and Hearing Services in Schools, 23,* 225–232.

Fisher, H., & Logemann, J. (1971). *Fisher-Logemann test of articulation competence.* Boston: Houghton-Mifflin.

Gierut, J. A. (1986). On the assessment of productive phonological knowledge. *Journal of the National Student Speech-Language-Hearing Association, 14,* 83–100.

Gierut, J. A., Elbert, M., & Dinnsen, D. A. (1986). Functional analysis of phonological knowledge and generalization learning in misarticulating children. *Journal of Speech and Hearing Research, 30,* 462–479.

Gierut, J.A., Morisette, M.L., Hughes, M.T., & Rowlands, S. (1996). Phonological treatment of efficacy and developmental norms. *Language, Speech, and Hearing Services in the Schools, 27,* 215–230.

Goldman, R., & Fristoe, M. (1986). *Goldman-Fristoe test of articulation.* Circle Pines, MN: American Guidance Service.

Grunwell, P. (1985). *Phonological assessment of child speech (PACS).* Windsor, UK: NFER-Nelson.

Grunwell, P. (1987). *Clinical phonology* (2nd ed.). Baltimore: Williams & Wilkins.

Grunwell, P. (1997). Developmental phonological disability: Order in disorder. In B. W. Hodson & M. L. Edwards (Eds.), *Perspectives in applied phonology* (pp. 61–103). Gaithersburg, MD: Aspen Publications.

Hodson, B. W. (1980). *Assessment of phonological processes.* Stonington, IL: PhonoComp.

Hodson, B. W. (1986). *Assessment of phonological processes-revised.* Austin, TX: Pro-Ed.

Hodson, B. W. (1992). Applied phonology: Constructs, contributions, and issues. Clinical forum: Phonological assessment and treatment. *Language, Speech, and Hearing Services in Schools, 23,* 247–253.

Ingram, D. (1976). *Phonological disability in children.* New York: American Elsevier.

Proctor, A. (1994). Phonology and cultural diversity. In R. J. Lowe (Ed.), *Phonology: Assessment and intervention applications in speech pathology* (207–245). Baltimore: Williams & Wilkins.

Sander, E. (1972). When are speech sounds learned? *Journal of Speech and Hearing Disorders, 37,* 55–63.

Shriberg, L. D., & Kwiatkowski, J. (1980). *Natural process analysis (NPA): A procedure for phonological analysis of continuous speech samples.* New York: John Wiley & Sons.

Stoel-Gammon, C. (1994). Early identification of phonological disorders. *Children's Phonology Disorders* (2nd ed.) (pp. 29–42). Rockville, MD: American Speech-Language-Hearing Association.

Stoel-Gammon, C. (1987). Phonological skills in 2-year-olds. *Language, Speech and Hearing Services in Schools, 18,* 323–329.

Turton, C. J. (1973). Diagnostic implications of articulation testing. In W. D. Wolfe & D. J. Goulding (Eds.), *Articulation and learning* (195–232). Springfield, IL: Charles C Thomas.

Weber, J.L. (1970). Patterning of deviant articulation behavior. *Journal of Speech and Hearing Disorders, 35,* 135–141.

Weiner, F. (1982). *Phonological process analysis.* Austin, TX.: Pro-Ed.

Williams, A. L. (1993). Phonological reorganization: A qualitative measure of phonological improvement. *American Journal of Speech-Language Pathology, 2,* 44–51.

Williams, A.L. (1998, October). *From assessment to intervention: Phonology principles to guide the SLP.* Workshop presented at the annual meeting of the Tennessee Association of Audiologists and Speech-Language Pathologists. Knoxville, TN.

APPENDIX 2.A   Phonological Process Analysis of Cameron's Single-Word Responses on the Goldman-Fristoe Test of Articulation

/tɛləfon/	**target**	/sɪzɚz/	**target**
tɛfon	WSD	sɪsɚs	DV-ll
dɛfon	PV	sɪtɚs	ST
[dɑfon]		[sɪʔɚs]	GR
/kʌp/	**target**	/dʌk/	**target**
kʌʔ	GR	[dʌʔ]	GR
tʌʔ	FR		
[sʌʔ]	idio	/jɛlo/	**target**
		[jɛʔo]	idio
/gʌn/	**target**		
dʌn	FR	/vækjum/	**target**
[dʌm]	idio	bækjum	ST
		[bæʔjum]	GR
/naɪf/	**target**		
[naɪ]	FCD	/mætʃəz/	**target**
		[mæʔəz]	DA+GR
/wɪndoʊ/	**target**		
wɪnoʊ	CR	/læmp/	**target**
wɪoʊ	CD	jæmp	GL
[wɛo]		[jæp]	CR
/wægən/	**target**	/ʃʌvəl/	**target**
[wædən]	FR	sʌvəl	FR
		sʌʔəl	idio
/tʃɪkən/	**target**	[sʌʔo]	vow
ʃɪkən	DA		
sɪkən	FR	/kar/	**target**
[sɪʔən]	GR	[sar]	idio
/zipɚ/	**target**	/ræbɪt/	**target**
[sipɚ]	DV	[ræʔɪt]	DV + GR
		/fɪʃɪŋ/	**target**
		[fɪʃɪŋ]	FR
/tʃɝtʃ/	**target**	/fiŋgɚ/	**target**
sɝtʃ	idio	figɚ	CR
[sɝts]	FR	fikɚ	DV
		[fiʔɚ]	GR
/fɛðɚ/	**target**		
[fɛʔɚ]	idio	/riŋ/	**target**
		wiŋ	GL

/pɪntsəlz/	target	[wi]	FCD				
p=ɪntsəlz	deasp.						
p=ɪtsəlz	CR	/dʒɑməz/	target				
[p=ɪʔsəlz]	GR	θɑməz	idio				
		[θɑməð]	FR				
/ðæt/	target						
dæt	ST			OR			
[dæʔ]	GR	/plen/	target		pwen	GL	
		pen	CR		wen	CR	
/kɛrɪt/	target	[fen]	idio		[fen]	LAB	
sɛrɪt	idio						
[sɛrɪʔ]	GR	/blu/	target				
		[bu]	CR				
/orɪndʒ/	target			OR			
ɔrɪdʒ	CR	/brʌʃ/	target		bwʌʃ	GL	
ɔrɪdz	FR	bʌʃ	CR		wʌʃ	CR	
[ɔrɪz]	DA	fʌʃ	idio		[fʌʃ]	LAB	
		[fʌθ]	FR		fʌθ	FR	
/bæətʌb/	target			OR			
bæʔtʌb	ST + GR	/drʌm/	target		dwʌm	GL	
[bæʔt=ʌb]	deasp.	dʌm	CR		wʌm	CR	
		[fʌm]	idio		[fʌm]	LAB	
/bæθ/	target						
[bæʔ]	ST + GR	/flæg/	target				
		fæg	CR				
/θʌm/	target	[fæ]	FCD				
[fʌm]	LAB						
/sænə klaz/	target						
θænə klað	FR-ǁ						
θæ˞klað	CD						
θæ˞kað	CR						
[θæ˞ θɑð]	assim.						
/krɪsməs tri/	target						
trɪsməs tri	FR						
trɪθməs tri	FR						
[trɪθ tri]	WSD						
/skwɝl/	target						
tɝl	CR						
[trʊl]	epen + vow						

		OR		
/slipɪŋ/	**target**			
lipɪŋ	CR		swipɪŋ	GL
fipɪŋ	idio		wipɪŋ	CR
[fipɪ]	FCD		fipɪŋ	LAB
			[fipɪ]	FCD
/bɛd/	**target**			
[bɛ]	FCD			
/stov/	**target**			
tov	CR			
[to]	FCD			

APPENDIX 2.B   Nonstandardized Phonological Process Analysis Summary Sheet

Clinician: _alw_____   Age: _____4-10_____

Structural Processes (Deletion)	Frequency of Occurrence $\left(\dfrac{\text{\#times occurred}}{\text{\# opportunities}} = \% \right)$	Approximate Age of Suppression (Grunwell, 1987)
Final Consonant Deletion (FCD)	6/33 = 18%	2:8
Initial Consonant Deletion (ICD)		
Cluster Reduction (CR)	14/21 = 67%	2:8 - 3:3
Weak Syllable Deletion (WSD)	2/8 = 25%	3:7
Consonant Deletion (CD)	2/17 = 12%	
Reduplication (RD)		2:1
Assimilation		
Labial Assimilation (LA)		
Nasal Assimilation (NA)		
Velar Assimilation (VA)		
Consonant Harmony (CH)	1/2 = 50%	2:4
Simplification Processes (Substitution)		
Stopping (ST)	5/30 = 17%	2:1 - 3:6
Fronting (FR)	14/26 = 54%	2:6
Gliding (GL)	6/8 = 75%	2:9
Vocalization (VO)	2/11 = 18%	
Deaffrication (DA)	3/7 = 43%	3:2
Apicalization (AP)		

Labalization (LB)	$5/5 = 100\%$	
Denasalization (DN)		
Glottal Replacement (GR)	16	
Palatalization (PL)		
Voicing (Voi)	$1/5 = 20\%$	2:4
Devoicing (DV)	$5/6 = 86\%$	2:4

Other Process

| Idiosyncratic Processes (IP) | $7\ [^s/_{k(3)};\ ^s/_{tʃ(2)};\ ^m/_{n(1)};\ ^\theta/_{dʒ(1)}]$ |
| Other | deaspiration-2 |

Summary

Classes of sounds/positions affected by processes:

FR (stops, affrics, frics) - wd initial   GR (stops, affrics) - wd medial   FCD (stops, frics) - wd final
                  CR - wd initial

Consistency of processes:

CR, GR - most consistent
IP, GL

Process interactions:

$$GR + < {ST \atop DA}$$

Persisting Normal Processes:

FR, CR, GL, FCD, ST

Idiosyncratic Processes:

$^s/_k;\ ^s/_{tʃ}$

APPENDIX 2.C   Place-Voice-Manner Error Pattern Analysis*

Place - Voice - Manner Error Pattern Analysis

Transcriber: __alw__

Error grid

Position	m	n	ŋ	p	b	t	d	k	g	θ	ð	f	v	s	z	ʃ	ʒ	h	tʃ	dʒ	l	r	w	j
Prevocalic #_	/	/	▓	pˀ	///	d tˀ	/	s-//	d	f	d	///	b	/ θ	s	s		/	s-// θ	θ	j	/ w	///	/
Intervocalic V_V	/	/	ø	~	~		~	~	d	~	~	/	~	~	~	s			~		ø ~	// ʊ		
Postvocalic _#	/	/// m	/ ø-//	~	/	/ ʔ-//	/ ø	~	ø	ʔ-//	ø	ø	ø	/ θ	s // ð-//	θ		▓	ts		/// o	/// ʔ-//	▓	▓
(Manner)	Nasals			Stops						Fricatives									Affricates		Liquids		Glides	

P.V.M. Error Patterns

__Place:__ palatals and velars replaced with alveolars

__Voice:__ V* consonants replaced by V glottal top V_V

__Manner:__ affricates and V* velar stop replaced with fricatives #____

__Other:__ Clusters replaced with singletons

Phonetic Inventory

```
p b   (t)(d)
f   (s) z   (ŋ)
m     n   (j)   (h)
w         l   r
```

Clusters

	/s/ clusters	/w/ clusters	/r/ clusters	/l/ clusters	nasal clusters
	tr/skw		f/br	f/pl	p/mp
	÷/st		f/dr	b/bl	z/ndʒ
		ʔj/kj	tr/kr	f/fl	ø/nd
			tr	θ/kl	ʔs/nts
				f/sl	ʔ/ŋg
	sm·sn·sp·st·sk	tw dw·kw·gw·sw	pr·br·tr·dr kr·gr·fr·ʃr·θr	pl·bl·kl·gl fl·sl	nt·nd·ndʒ·mp

---

*Reprinted with permission from Elbert, M., & Gierut, J. A. (1986). *Handbook of Clinical Phonology: Approaches to Assessment and Treatment.* San Diego: College Hill Press.

APPENDIX 2.D Systemic Phonological Analysis

Clinician: __alw__   Age: ____4-10____

I.   *Phonetic Inventory (Systemic)*

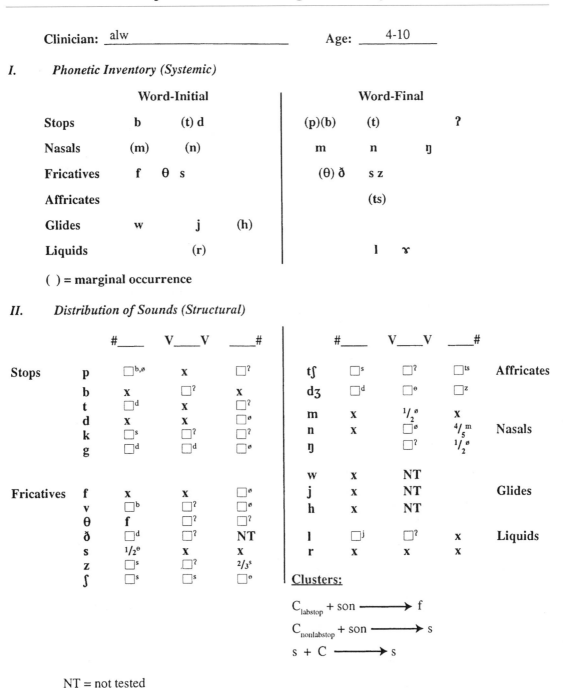

	Word-Initial				Word-Final		
Stops	b	(t) d		(p)(b)	(t)		**ʔ**
Nasals	(m)	(n)		m	n	ŋ	
Fricatives	f θ s			(θ) ð	s z		
Affricates					(ts)		
Glides	w	j	(h)				
Liquids		(r)			l ɚ		

( ) = marginal occurrence

II.   *Distribution of Sounds (Structural)*

		#___	V___V	___#
Stops	p	☐b,ø	x	☐ʔ
	b	x	☐ʔ	x
	t	☐d	x	☐ʔ
	d	x	x	☐ø
	k	☐s	☐ʔ	☐ʔ
	g	☐d	☐d	☐ø
Fricatives	f	x	x	☐ø
	v	☐b	☐ʔ	☐ø
	θ	f	☐ʔ	☐ʔ
	ð	☐d	☐ʔ	NT
	s	1/2ᵉ	x	x
	z	☐s	☐ʔ	2/3ˢ
	ʃ	☐s	☐s	☐ᵉ

		#___	V___V	___#	
Affricates	tʃ	☐s	☐ʔ	☐ts	
	dʒ	☐d	☐ᵉ	☐z	
Nasals	m	x	¹/₂ ø	x	
	n	x	☐ø	⁴/₅ m	
	ŋ		☐ʔ	¹/₂ ø	
Glides	w	x	NT		
	j	x	NT		
	h	x	NT		
Liquids	l	☐j	☐ʔ	x	
	r	x	x	x	

Clusters:

$C_{labstop}$ + son ⟶ f

$C_{nonlabstop}$ + son ⟶ s

s + C ⟶ s

NT = not tested

III. Mapping Child-to-Adult Systems (Phoneme Collapses)

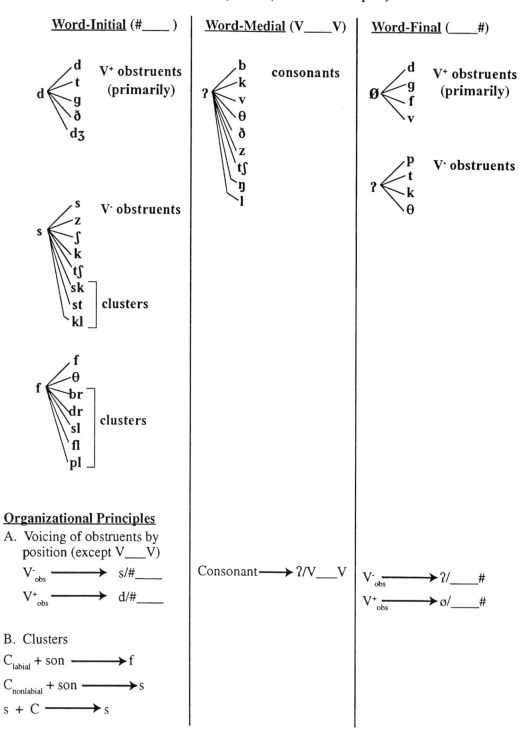

Organizational Principles

Word-Initial (#___)

Word-Medial (V___V)

Word-Final (___#)

A. Voicing of obstruents by position (except V___V)

$V^-_{obs} \longrightarrow s/\#\_\_\_\_$

$V^+_{obs} \longrightarrow d/\#\_\_\_\_$

Consonant $\longrightarrow$?/V___V

$V^-_{obs} \longrightarrow$?/____#

$V^+_{obs} \longrightarrow$ ø/____#

B. Clusters

C_{labial} + son $\longrightarrow$ f

$C_{nonlabial}$ + son $\longrightarrow$ s

s + C $\longrightarrow$ s

3 Language Assessment during Childhood

Ronald B. Gillam
LaVae M. Hoffman

Critical Issues in Assessment and Identification

Our view of language impairment is based on the most recent version of the International Classification of Functioning and Disability (ICIDH-2) from the World Health Organization (WHO) (World Health Organization, 1999), which was in beta form as this chapter was being written. Currently, WHO defines an impairment as a temporary or permanent deviation from generally accepted standards. Deviations must adversely affect one of three dimensions: physiologic or psychological structures and functions, the ability to perform activities (life tasks), or participation in life situations.

In this chapter, we advocate for what Tomblin et al. (1996) and Fey (1988) have called the *normativist approach* to the assessment and identification of language disorders in children. The hallmark of this approach is the idea that *disabilities* or *impairments* (we use those terms interchangeably) should be viewed with respect to social and cultural values and expectations. We combined the normativist perspective and the revised WHO classification of functioning and disability to create the following definition of childhood language impairment in children.

A child has a language impairment when he or she presents one or more of the following:

- Significant difficulties with the underlying cognitive or linguistic structures and functions that support language learning
- Limitations in language form, content, or use that interfere with age-appropriate participation in important social or educational activities

TABLE 3.1 Areas of assessment related to the International Classification of Functioning and Disability from the World Health Organization

Psychological functions (competence)	Communication activities (performance/use)	Participation (level of involvement)	Environmental factors (supports/hindrances)
Attention: sustaining, shifting, dividing	Basic learning activities: spontaneous learning situations	Family activities: involvement in activities that occur at home	Products for communication: equipment or systems that affect participation
Perception: discriminating tones, sounds, and words	Conversation activities: conversing with relatives, friends, and strangers	Social relationships: involvement in friendships and acceptance by neighbors	Family support: individuals and organizations that influence beliefs and values
Memory: working, long-term, executive functions	Interpersonal activities: interacting with relatives, friends, and strangers	Education settings: involvement in school situations	Friends: peers who affect participation and influence beliefs and values
Reception of language: understanding spoken, written, or signed messages	Preschool/school activities: formal educational experiences with groups of children and a teacher	Religion and spirituality: involvement in religious or spiritual activities	Caregivers/teachers: individuals who affect participation
Expression of language: producing meaningful messages in spoken, written, or signed forms	Recreational activities: play, organized games, art, crafts, hobbies	Recreation and leisure: involvement in sports, games, art activities, crafts	Individual attitudes and beliefs that affect participation
Reasoning/problem-solving: solving problems by forming conclusions, inferences, or judgments	—	—	—

Source: Ronald B. Gillam, Ph.D., Jesse H. Jones Communication Center, Austin, Texas. Copyright © 2000.

- Limitations in language form, content, or use that place the child at risk for restricted participation in important social or educational activities in the future

Assessment should provide speech-language pathologists (SLPs) with the information they need to evaluate children's psychological structures underlying language development (attention, perception, memory, reasoning), their knowledge of language structure and functions, their engagement in communication activities, and their participation in important experiences (Table 3.1).

SLPs are not trained to assess physiological structures related to language (the ear and the nervous system) beyond routine screening. However, SLPs can assess many psychological functions that support language development, communication activities, and participation in areas of life that are important to the child's social and cultural community. These functions include attention, perception, memory, receptive language, expressive language, and reasoning. There are four primary ways to determine whether children have significant difficulties with underlying cognitive or linguistic structures and functions: (1) administration of information processing tasks and measures, (2) language sample analysis, (3) dynamic assessment, and (4) standardized testing. Clinicians should also assess participation in activities, the child's level of involvement in social, educational, and prevocational experiences, and environmental factors that hinder or facilitate functioning and participation. These areas are best assessed by interviewing children, parents, and teachers and by observing children in their natural environments.

Cultural Considerations

Language is, by its very nature, inseparable from culture. Language is a vehicle through which exchanges occur both within and between cultures, and languages are embodiments of cultural norms, perspectives, and values. It is difficult to become truly familiar with a language without learning also about the culture in which the language functions. To judge whether a child presents a temporary or permanent deviation from generally accepted language standards, it is necessary to understand the norms and expectations of the cultural environment in which the child is developing.

For example, mainstream American adults often ask questions to which they obviously know the answer as a means of prompting children to display their knowledge. Children in mainstream American culture are familiar with this routine and respond in a straightforward fashion, often with some degree of pride in their ability to answer correctly. This is not necessarily a valid interactive exchange in all cultures. Some cultures would find this type of a verbal exchange to be meaningless or even absurd, and a child who is being raised in such a culture would most likely find it very awkward to respond to an adult who has such a limited grasp of the obvious so as to ask "What is this?" as they hold up a simple object. During assessment, children from diverse cultures may demonstrate responses, behaviors, or skills that do not coincide with the expectations of the examiner. The critical question becomes: At what point is the child demonstrating a language disorder as opposed to a language difference? When assessing the language development of children from cultures that are different from the examiner's, it is vital that the examiner become as familiar as possible with the cultural factors that create the language milieu of the child as well as their own cultural orientation.

Published materials can be an important resource for the SLP, but these should never be relied on to the exclusion of personal networking within the community being served. It is important to keep in mind that the diagnosis of a language disorder must come from within the perspective of the culture that is raising the child. It should never be superimposed externally by an SLP, no matter how well intentioned.

It is impossible to be culture-free. Assessment instruments and methods are cultural phenomena. Further, no examiner is free of cultural bias and background. The extensive training SLPs undergo is culturally based, and the resulting ability to interpret children's development is founded on the explicit refinement and reification of cultural expectations, usually those of the mainstream culture. To further complicate the issue, it could be said that the observation of a child's language abilities in the presence of the examiner reflects the child's skills and abilities on that particular day in that particular context while interacting with a professional of whatever age, culture, gender, and disposition that the child perceives that examiner to be. Within the complex mix of language, culture, human development, and variability, how can any examiner hope to obtain valid assessment results? By being as knowledgeable about cultural issues as possible, by maintaining professional standards of ethical practices, and by relying on the input and perception of others who interact with the child on an ongoing basis. No single professional has to be thoroughly familiar with all cultures, but every professional must know how to draw on resources to provide the information needed when appropriate.

A Framework for Assessment

Figure 3.1 represents our assessment framework. Imagine that the circle represents the entire assessment process. When evaluating infants and toddlers, the assessment process should consist of observation of functions, activities, and participation. When evaluating preschool and school-age children, SLPs should allocate a considerable amount of their assessment efforts to observation, but they should also administer contextualized and decontextualized measures. Clinicians can observe language and psychological functions when they collect and analyze samples of conversation and narration or when they conduct dynamic assessments. Clinicians can observe *how* children use language when they watch children communicate in their daily environments. Clinicians can observe parent and teacher perceptions of *underlying processes* and *what* children say when they conduct interviews.

For preschool and school-age children, the other half of one's assessment time should be spent administering, scoring, and interpreting contextualized and decontextualized measures of activities and participation. Contextualized measures for school-age children include criterion-referenced curriculum measures and reading miscue inventories. Decontextualized measures for preschool and school-age children include standardized tests that assess underlying psycholinguistic functions or language activities.

Observation of Language Functions and Activities

We believe observation is the most critical aspect of assessment. Too often, we have worked with colleagues who allocated 90% of their assessment time to standardized testing and only 10% of their assessment time to observation. These clinicians did not gather the informa-

Observation

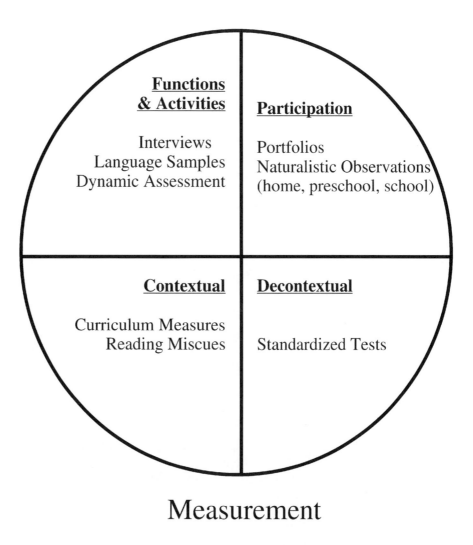

**Functions
& Activities**

Interviews
Language Samples
Dynamic Assessment

Participation

Portfolios
Naturalistic Observations
(home, preschool, school)

Contextual

Curriculum Measures
Reading Miscues

Decontextual

Standardized Tests

Measurement

FIGURE 3.1   *Assessment framework. (Ronald B. Gillam, Ph.D., Jesse H. Jones
Communication Center, Austin, Texas. Copyright © 2000.)*

tion they needed for a comprehensive language evaluation. Careful
observation, description, and analysis enable clinicians to capture and
clarify parents' and teachers' expectations for communication and children's ability to meet those expectations. As noted by Silliman and
Wilkinson (1994), observation involves more that watching children talk
and play. Like Silliman and Wilkinson, we view observation as a method

of inquiry that incorporates interviews, language samples, and dynamic assessment as the means for assessing psycholinguistic functions and activities.

Interviews

Parent and teacher interviews provide important information about children's language abilities and their participation in culturally relevant communication contexts. We have created a parent interview (Appendix 3.A) that is based on the revised WHO classification of functioning and disability (World Health Organization, 1999). Our interview procedure was strongly influenced by Westby (1990), who explains that professionals need to discover how children are viewed with respect to their culture. The interview in Appendix 3.A contains many general questions that are designed to elicit descriptions of psychological functions, communication activities, participation in daily events, and environmental factors that support or hinder communication. We recommend conducting parent interviews in person or by phone before children are assessed. Many of the questions we ask parents are also appropriate for teachers.

Language Samples

Language analysis has long been a mainstay of speech-language assessment. Guidelines for collecting and analyzing language samples have been described in depth (see Cole et al., 1989; Dollaghan & Campbell, 1992; Dunn et al., 1996; Evans, 1996; Evans & Craig, 1992; Kemp & Klee, 1997; Leadholm & Miller, 1992; Stockman, 1996). The beginning clinician should be thoroughly familiar with these publications. In essence, a language sample should be collected in a setting that is as familiar to the child as possible, with materials that prompt verbal exchanges. We use Leadholm and Miller's language sampling protocol for collecting conversation and narrative samples from children between the ages of 3 and 13 years (Appendix 3.B). Clinicians should also familiarize themselves with Hadley's (1998) useful step-by-step procedures for collecting conversation and narrative samples from school-age children. Her language sampling suggestions are based on the Leadholm and Miller protocol. Language samples should be audio- or videotaped and transcribed for later analysis.

The required length of the language sample has been debated within the field, with authors suggesting ranges from 50 to 200 child utterances. It is our opinion that the number of utterances you collect and analyze is, in large part, dependent on the quality of the sample obtained and the intended analytic procedures. SLPs should thoroughly sample the structures and functions they are interested in evaluating. In most situations, a 15- to 20-minute sample of conversation and narration should elicit between 75 and 150 utterances from the child. This should be sufficient for beginning the language analysis process.

Computer language analysis systems have been developed to assist in the always laborious and often tedious process of analyzing language samples. After a language sample transcript is keyed in and coded, these

TABLE 3.2 Some of the measures that can be obtained from the Systematic Analysis of Language Transcripts (SALT) profiler

	Score	± SD
Total utterances		
MLU		
Type-token ratio		
Number different word roots		
Total main body words		
Mean turn length		
Responses to questions		
Yes/no responses to questions		
Percent intelligible utterances		
Utterances with mazes		
Number of mazes		
Number of maze words		
Percent of maze words/total words		
Utterances with overlaps		
Number of complete words		
Elapsed time		
Utterances/minute		
Words/minute		
Between utterances pauses		
Between utterance pause time		
Within utterance pauses		
Within utterance pause time		
Omitted words		
Omitted bound morphemes		
Abandoned utterances		
Word-level error codes		
Utterance-level error codes		

programs can quickly calculate analyses that would take the clinician a considerable length of time. Our favorite language analysis program is Systematic Analysis of Language Transcripts (SALT) (Miller & Chapman, 1998), which comes with a database for comparing a number of language measures with same-age children from Wisconsin. The profiler provides information about the mean and standard deviation for each measure as well as a z score, which indicates how many standard deviations the child's score on each measure falls from the mean for his or her comparison group. A few of the measures in the profile are listed in Table 3.2.

We provide a step-by-step procedure for analyzing and coding language samples in Appendix 3.C. Clinicians who do not have the resources

TABLE 3.3   Characteristics of dynamic assessment

Dynamic assessment is interactive. In contrast to traditional static approaches in which examiners observe children in a more neutral manner, examiners using dynamic assessment become an active part of the assessment. Examiners observe and interpret observations on line to facilitate change and to reveal learning.

Dynamic assessment focuses on the learning process. During mediated teaching, examiners focus on how children solve problems and how children learn. Observations reveal information about children's learning strategies and the amount of effort required for learning new skills.

Dynamic assessment yields information about learner responsiveness. Examiners make judgments about how easily children respond to new teaching and how well new strategies are incorporated into performance.

Source: Ronald B. Gillam, Ph.D. and Elizabeth D. Peña, Ph.D., Jesse H. Jones Communication Center, Austin, Texas. Copyright © 1999.

to purchase the SALT program can still compare a child's language sample measures to the SALT database, which is published in *Language Sample Analysis: The Wisconsin Guide* (Leadholm & Miller, 1992).

Dynamic Assessment

Dynamic assessment enables SLPs to observe psychological and linguistic functions and activities as children are involved in language learning. Dynamic assessment is a test-teach-retest procedure that can be used with nearly any formal or informal task. Dynamic assessment usually begins with a testing phase in which the examiner administers a pretest. During a teaching phase, the examiner teaches one or two lessons that are designed to affect the child's performance on the pretest measure. Then, in the post-test phase, examiners readminister the pretest. Important characteristics of dynamic assessment are summarized in Table 3.3.

Dynamic assessment yields data about language-learning functions and language-learning potential. Children's responses to the teaching phase of dynamic assessment provide important data about attention, perception, and memory functions during language learning. The amount and type of changes that result from intervention are an indication of language-learning potential.

Researchers (Gillam et al., 1999; Miller et al., 2000; Peña & Gillam, 2000) have described a detailed approach for the dynamic assessment of narratives. We begin by having children create stories as they look through wordless picture books. Then we mediate some aspect of storytelling in two separate intervention sessions. After the mediation sessions, we ask children to create a story about a second wordless picture book that contains the same number of pictures and the same story structure as the book that was used for the pretest.

We use two wordless picture books: *Two Friends* (Miller, 2000a) for collecting the pretest narrative and *Bird and His Ring* (Miller, 2000b) for collecting the post-test narrative. Children are invited to look through the

TABLE 3.4 Narrative analyses

Story productivity

    Total number of words

    Total number of C-units

    Total number of clauses

    Number of clauses per C-unit

Episode structure

    Incomplete episode—one or two story elements (initiating event, internal response, plan, attempt, consequence, reaction/ending)

    Basic episode (initiating event, attempt, and consequence)

    Basic episode plus one element

    Basic episode plus two elements

    Complete episode

    Multiple episode story

Story components

    Setting (references to time and place)

    Character information (descriptions of the characters)

    Temporal order (use of adverbial phrases and clauses to clarify the sequence of events)

    Causal relationships (explanations about the reasons for the events in a story)

Story ideas and language

    Complexity of ideas (the concreteness or abstractness of the ideas in a story)

    Complexity of vocabulary (elaborateness of the vocabulary)

    Grammatical complexity (use of compound and complex sentences)

    Dialogue (use of character dialogue)

    Creativity (elements that make stories interesting and captivating)

Source: Lynda Miller, Ph.D., SMART Alternatives, Austin, Texas; Ronald B. Gillam, Ph.D. and Elizabeth D. Peña, Ph.D., Jesse H. Jones Communication Center, Austin, Texas. Copyright © 1999.

book without saying anything to formulate a story that corresponds with the sequence of pictures in the book. Then they return to the beginning and tell the part of the story that goes with each page. We prompt them with, "Is that all that happens there?" or "Tell me what is happening here" if they are unusually reticent or skip pages.

The stories are audiotaped and transcribed into C-units (units consisting of the main clause and all subordinated clauses; Appendix 3.D) (Hunt, 1965). We analyze the pre- and post-test stories for language productivity analyses (number of words, number of C-units, number of clauses, and number of clauses per C-unit), episode structure, story components, and story ideas and language. The various components of our story analysis strategy are summarized in Table 3.4.

We select the goals for the two mediation sessions based on our analysis of the pretest story. We usually select two aspects of narration from two different areas of our analysis scheme. We target aspects of narration that the child has some knowledge of in one of our mediation sessions. For example, if a child's story contained an incomplete episode, we might decide to focus on teaching a missing element that would be required for a basic episode (initiating event, attempt, or consequence). During the second mediation session, we usually target an aspect of narration that the child did not demonstrate any knowledge of. For example, we might focus on information about the setting if the child did not include any information about where the story occurred.

We begin our mediation sessions by explaining the learning goal to clarify the purpose of the lesson. Next, we explain why that goal is important. For instance, if a child's story did not contain a basic episode, we would tell him or her that the purpose of the lesson was to learn about telling stories, and that the focus was on telling the listener what the problem of the story was (the initiating event). We would explain that good storytellers tell their listeners what the main problem in the story is. That makes the story interesting and lets the listeners know why the characters are acting the way they are.

Next, we help the child associate the goal of the lesson to other events that might be more familiar to him or her. The examiner may use "what if" questions to help the child understand the goal, its importance, and its relevance to other daily life situations. For example, the examiner might ask, "What if you wanted to ride your bike to your friend's house, but the tires were flat. What would you do?" If your child said something like, "I'd pump them up with air," the examiner could say, "Yes, then they wouldn't be flat anymore, would they? The problem is that the tires were flat. When you pumped them up with air, you solved the problem. Stories are like that. People usually say what the problem was, what someone did to try to solve it, and how it was solved. So, today, we're going to talk about telling listeners what the problem is."

Then, we work through some examples. We often start with the *Two Friends* story because it a simple story that the child has had recent experience with. However, any simple children's story with a clear problem works fine. We work through a storytelling with the child, repeatedly emphasizing what the problem is and reminding the child to restate the problem, the actions taken to solve it, and the solution. After we create a story together, we ask the child to tell a story without our help, reminding him or her to be sure to include a problem (the initiating event), actions taken to solve the problem (attempts), and the solution to the problem (the consequence). We often prompt the child to tell us a familiar folk tale, such as "Goldilocks and the Three Bears" or "The Three Little Pigs."

Once the child creates a basic episode story without our help, we talk to the child about creating a plan for using what he or she just learned. We may help the child develop strategies, such as making a story map to identify the "problem" in a story. Often, children tell us what they think about the *Two Friends* story, and that helps them remember to tell about the problem. After two of these sessions, we rate the amount of the teacher effort that was needed to help the child improve as well as the level of the child's responsiveness to teaching. We also note which strategies appeared to be the most helpful for the child.

We administer a post-test after two mediation sessions. We follow the same procedure for analyzing and describing the post-test story that was used for analyzing and describing the pretest story. We consider the kinds of changes the child made, how much effort was required to accomplish these changes, and the type of the change that was observed. More specifically, we ask

- Was the child able to form a more complete or more coherent story after mediation?
- How hard did the SLP have to work for the child to make positive changes?
- Did the child attend well and stay on task?
- Once the SLP's support was withdrawn (as in the second story), was the child able to transfer what he or she learned to his or her own story?
- Was the child's learning quick and efficient or slow and labored?

The answers to these question are useful for determining whether a child's underlying psycholinguistic functions are sufficient to support language learning. Children who make rapid changes and who are highly responsive to the mediation sessions rarely have language disorders. These children, when provided with instruction that focuses their attention on the necessary elements of narratives, are able to quickly and efficiently make changes. On the other hand, children who need continued support and who have a very difficult time making even small changes, are very likely to have a language impairment. These children typically demonstrate low responsiveness, require high examiner effort, and demonstrate few pre- to post-test changes.

Observation of Participation

Language is a generative, dynamic process that occurs in many contexts and with many conversational partners. SLPs should observe children in their natural communication settings to determine what communicative activities they participate in and what their level of participation is. Home and classroom observations create records of children's transitory, interpersonal, and verbal processes. These static glimpses of how children use language to function in their world can provide the SLP with valuable evidence of impairment. In the hands of a skilled clinician, products of language use can be analyzed and evaluated to support diagnosis, intervention goals, and intervention procedures. Checklists, narrative records, and portfolios are useful tools for assessing and recording the level of the child's participation in everyday activities.

Naturalistic Observations

Home
When we assess toddlers and preschool-aged children, we often go to their homes to observe them as they play with their parents and siblings. If we are assessing preschoolers in an educational setting, we observe

children as they are playing with their peers. When our assessments are conducted in a clinical setting, we ask the parents to play with their children for a while at the very beginning of the assessment process. We invite parents to play with their children using some of their children's favorite toys as well as some toys we provide. Following Wetherby and Prizant (1992), we encourage parents not to tell their children what to do. Rather, we ask that they wait for their children to begin playing and then respond naturally. We advise using the following set of materials, which usually occupies parents and children for approximately 20 minutes:

- One of the child's favorite toys from home
- A simple windup toy
- Bubbles
- Three age-appropriate books (from home or from the clinic)
- A plush toy, automotive garage, zoo, or farm toy set

When we observe children, we look for the communication behaviors provided in a checklist by Dickson et al. (1997). They suggest clinicians should observe children's communicative intentions, gestures, communicative functions, discourse skills, sound production patterns, semantic relationships, sentence structure, morphologic markers, comprehension of language, oral motor development, voice quality, cognitive development, and social-emotional development (Appendix 3.E).

Classroom Communication
Patterson and Gillam (1995) created a form for observing language use in classroom contexts (Appendix 3.F). Clinicians observe the child who has been referred for assessment as well as another child who is functioning well within the normal range. Clinicians can code children's utterances for assertive and responsive utterances (Fey, 1988) and utterance level discourse functions, such as topic maintenance, syntactic acceptability, or semantic acceptability. We usually observe children during a part of the school day that has been set aside for small group interaction (e.g., reading centers or science labs). We try to code approximately 10 minutes of communication that includes the student who was referred for assessment and a student whom the teacher believes to be an average communicator.

Portfolios

Samples of the children's homework, class assignments, tests, and writing folders can provide the opportunity to observe the ability to use language to meet the expectations and demands of academic contexts. Children can be asked to review their homework assignments, tests, and writing folders with the SLP. After a classroom observation or language sample, we often ask children about their participation in classroom activities and their perceptions about their success. Statements from the child about areas of difficulty and learning strategies they use can reveal important information about their language functioning.

Clinicians should have a good understanding of the teacher's performance expectations for the class. SLPs and classroom teachers can collaborate to investigate children's areas of language difficulty using products of language that are readily at hand in most classrooms: homework assignments, participation in reading groups, and written stories. Information of this type should be reviewed both within and across content areas to determine whether there are communication difficulties that are specific to certain topics or instructional activities. Clinicians and teachers should also look for stable characteristics of the child's language form, function, and use. It is important also to examine classroom materials to assess strengths as well as weaknesses. Questions to consider while investigating these language products are listed in Appendix 3.G.

Contextual Measurements

Curriculum Measures

Children are tested repeatedly in today's schools. Many states have instituted tests to determine which children can graduate from high school and which children can be promoted to the next grade. We believe these tests are often misused for political purposes, and the results are nearly always overinterpreted. SLPs need to take an interest in state-mandated tests, however, because these tests provide another piece of information about children's level of participation in school activities.

Some schools administer tests that are designed to assess how well children perform with respect to the district's curriculum standards. These criterion-referenced or "benchmark" tests (children's scores are compared with curricular expectations rather than with state or national norms) can be useful for determining what the formal language expectations of the curriculum are and how well the child meets those expectations.

Reading Miscues

Children with language impairments often present difficulties with reading (Gillam, 1990; Gillam & Carlile, 1997; Tallal et al., 1997). Analysis of oral reading can provide information about students' reading strategies and their ability to use language for an academic task. One useful procedure for collecting and analyzing samples of oral reading is the Reading Miscue Inventory (RMI) (Goodman et al., 1987). In this procedure, children read stories aloud and then retell them. Examiners analyze the nature of the discrepancies between the author's text and the words the child reads. These discrepancies (referred to as *miscues*) are scored for graphophonemic, syntactic, and semantic-pragmatic similarity to the author's intended text. We do not use this assessment to evaluate reading, although it can be useful for that. Rather, we administer the RMI to assess how children use their language knowledge during a literacy task. We leave the evaluation of reading skills to diagnosticians, special education teachers, and reading specialists.

Story retelling is also part of the RMI procedure. Story retelling provides students with the opportunity to use their own language to reflect on and repeat the story they just read. Retellings reveal how students modify and integrate the story's vocabulary, language, and propositions into their own narratives. This procedure also provides data for comparing reading abilities and spoken language abilities.

To elicit reading miscues, examiners ask children to read short stories that are approximately one grade level above their measured reading level. First, students are given a book that is opened to their story and are asked to read the story aloud. They are informed that they will be asked to retell the story in their own words after reading it. They are also informed that the examiner cannot assist them with deciphering words as they read. Once they start reading, all the examiner can do is encourage them to continue when they stop, lose their place, or perseverate on a particular word.

Each reading and retelling is audio-recorded for later analysis. Typed scripts of the texts of the stories are marked for reader substitutions, omissions, insertions, repetitions, and corrections according to RMI conventions (Goodman et al., 1987) (Appendix 3.H).

For a gross indicator of word identification during oral reading, we determine the percentage of total words that are miscued. This is calculated by dividing the total number of miscues by the total number of words in the story, then multiplying that dividend by 100. To evaluate self-monitoring during reading, we calculated the percentage of miscues that were self-corrected by each student. Students who are aware of their reading and are monitoring themselves as they read often have 15% or more self-corrections.

Graphophonemic Analysis

Each substitution miscue is judged for its graphophonemic similarity to the author-intended word. For this study, graphophonemic similarity refers to the similarity between the phoneme sequence of the miscue in comparison with the graphically represented phoneme sequence of the written word. A miscue that retains between 66% and 100% of the phoneme sequence of the original word is classified as "high" in graphophonemic similarity. A miscue that retains between 33% and 65% of the phoneme sequence of the original word is classified as having "some" graphophonemic similarity. A miscue that retains less than 33% of the phonemes in the original word is classified as having "little" graphophonemic similarity. If a child read *string* for *sheet*, this miscue would be classified as having little graphophonemic similarity. Readers who are having many difficulties with phonics and sound blending often have high percentages (30% or higher) of miscues with little or some graphophonic similarity.

Syntactic Analysis

Sentences containing one or more uncorrected miscues are evaluated for syntactic acceptability. Self-corrected miscues are ignored, much like mazes in oral language are ignored in judgments of syntactic and semantic-pragmatic acceptability. Sentences containing miscues that interfere with grammaticality are judged to be syntactically unacceptable. Sentences without miscues were not included in the analysis because the intent was to determine the extent to which miscues interfered with syntax. In children with syntactic problems, we often find that 20% or more of their sentences containing a miscue are syntactically unacceptable.

Semantic-Pragmatic Analysis

The meaning of sentences containing uncorrected miscues is compared with the evaluator's understanding of the authors' intended meaning. When the reader's sentences are semantically and pragmatically related to the authors' sentences, they are judged to have no meaning change. When minor concepts, events, or characters are omitted or altered as a result of reader miscues, sentences are judged to reflect partial meaning changes. When important concepts, events, or characters are omitted or altered, sentences are judged to reflect significant meaning changes. For example, if the text was, "The cow crossed the road," but the student read, "The car covered the road," the sentence would be scored as syntactically acceptable because *car* and *cow* are both nouns, and *covered* and *crossed* are both verbs. If the sentence was part of a story about cows, and crossing the road was an important event in the story, this miscue would represent an important change to the author's intended meaning and would be classified as a significant meaning change.

Retelling Analyses

Story retellings are analyzed for their consistency with the original stories. We look to see whether children include all the important participants in the story in their retelling and provide basic setting (time and place) information. We also look to see if the child has included the initiating event, any important character responses to the initiating event, the critical actions, the consequences of those actions, any reactions to the consequences, and an ending.

Three measures are calculated to determine how closely each student's retelling follows the original story. Retention of specific vocabulary is evaluated by calculating the percentage of word roots from the original story that are retained in the retelling. Retention of story structure is evaluated by calculating the percentage of original story constituents (setting, initiating events, internal responses, plans, attempts, consequences, reactions, and endings) that were retained in the retelling. Gillam and Carlile (1997) provide specific examples of this miscue and retelling analysis system.

Contextual measures are normed and criterion-referenced tests of school performance. These measures can yield important information about the level of children's performance on activities related to language development. Many clinicians also administer decontextualized (context-free) standardized tests. We believe clinicians should not allocate more than 25% of their total assessment time to administering and scoring standardized tests.

Decontextualized Measurement

Many clinicians think of standardized testing as the primary component of language assessment. We place a discussion of standardized testing last because we believe it is the least important and least valuable component of assessment. This is because the items on most standardized tests of language are far removed from contextual language. Unfortunately, too many administrators in public education settings and in medical settings have the misguided perception that performance on standardized tests is the gold standard for determining whether a child presents a deviation from generally accepted standards. Test scores can be informative when a well-trained examiner administers a well-standardized test to a child who is a member of the author's culture and the culture of the majority of the children in the standardization sample. However, many of the children we test are not members of the mainstream cultural group (but the vast majority of test authors are), and none of the language tests we know of meets the majority of the standards for educational and psychological testing established by the American Educational Research Association, the American Psychological Association, and National Council on Measurement in Education (1985).

The culture of educational testing and health care in the United States is strongly supportive of standardized testing. We believe standardized tests should be used judiciously. If clinicians feel they must give a norm-referenced test, we recommend that they give only one or two tests. A number of the more popular standardized tests are listed in Table 3.5.

Some of the tests listed in Table 3.5 are useful for obtaining particular kinds of information. To gain an impression of the parent's perception of communication and socialization, we recommend the Vineland Adaptive Behavior Scales (Sparrow et al., 1984). To assess general linguistic skills underlying language development in preschoolers, we recommend the Clinical Evaluation of Language Fundamentals—Preschool (Wiig et al., 1992) or the Preschool Language Scale—3 (Zimmerman et al., 1992). To assess psycholinguistic skills underlying language development in school-age children, we recommend the Clinical Evaluation of Language Fundamentals (Semel et al., 1996), the Detroit Tests of Learning Aptitude (Hammill, 1998), or the Comprehensive Test of Phonological Processing (Wagner et al., 1999). To assess general language skills in school-age children, we recommend the Oral and Written Language Scales (Carrow-Woolfolk, 1995) or the Test of Language Development—Primary (Newcomer & Hammill, 1997). Finally, to gain a general indication of language skills in adolescents, we recommend the Test of Adolescent and Adult Language (Hammill, 1994). There are many other suitable language tests on the market. This is simply a list of the ones we use ourselves.

We encourage clinicians to always report the obtained deviation quotients and the 68% confidence intervals (one standard error of measurement) around those quotients. To do this, clinicians simply add one standard error of measurement to the obtained deviation quotient and subtract one standard error of measurement from the obtained score. Clinicians can be confident that 68% of the time, the child's true score will fall in this range. Reporting confidence intervals shows that clinicians understand the nature of error in standardized testing. As recommended by McCauley and Swisher (1984), clinicians should avoid reporting age scores (they are the least reliable and informative type of score), avoid basing conclusions about strengths and weaknesses of the child's perfor-

TABLE 3.5   Some frequently used standardized tests

Test name	Author	Age range (years; months)	Subtests
Clinical Evaluation of Language Fundamentals, 3rd Edition	Semel, Wiig, & Secord (1996)	6;0–21;11	Receptive language: sentence structure, concepts and directions, word classes
			Expressive language: word structure, formulated sentences, recalling sentences, sentence assembly
			Supplementary subtests: listening to paragraphs, word associations
Clinical Evaluation of Language Fundamentals—Preschool	Wiig, Secord, & Semel (1992)	3;0–6;11	Receptive language: recalling linguistic concepts, basic concepts, sentence structure
			Expressive language: sentences in context, formulating labels, word structure
Comprehensive Test of Phonological Processing	Wagner, Torgeson, & Rashotte (1999)	5;0–24;11	Phonological awareness: elision, blending words, sound matching, blending nonwords, phoneme reversal, segmenting words, segmenting nonwords
			Phonological memory: memory for digits, nonword repetition
			Rapid naming: rapid color naming, rapid letter naming, rapid object naming
Detroit Tests of Learning Aptitude, 4th Edition	Hammill (1998)	6;0–17;11	Verbal composite: word opposites, sentence imitation, story construction, basic information, word sequences
			Nonverbal composite: design sequences, design reproduction, reversed letters, symbolic relations, story sequences
Oral and Written Language Scales: Listening Comprehension and Oral Expression	Carrow-Woolfolk (1995)	3;0–21;11	Listening comprehension (includes items addressing semantics, syntax, figurative language, inferencing, pragmatics)
			Oral expression (includes items measuring semantics, syntax, figurative language, inferencing, and pragmatics)
Oral and Written Language Scales: Written Expression Scale	Carrow-Woolfolk (1995)	5;0–21;11	Writing conventions, semantics, syntax, discourse
Preschool Language Scale, 3rd Edition	Zimmerman, Steiner, & Pond (1992)	0;0–6;11	Auditory comprehension (includes items addressing semantics, syntax, and morphology)
			Expressive communication (includes items addressing semantics, syntax, morphology, and pragmatics)
Test of Adolescent and Adult Language	Hammill, Brown, Larsen, & Wiederholt (1994)	12;0–24;11	Listening: vocabulary, grammar Speaking: vocabulary, grammar Reading: vocabulary, grammar Writing: vocabulary, grammar

TABLE 3.5   continued

Test name	Author	Age range (years; months)	Subtests
Test of Language Development—Primary, 3rd Edition	Newcomer & Hammill (1997)	4;0–8;11	Vocabulary: picture vocabulary, relational vocabulary, oral vocabulary
			Grammar: grammatic understanding, sentence imitation, grammatic completion
			Supplemental: word articulation, phonemic analysis, word discrimination
Vineland Adaptive Behavior Scales	Sparrow, Balla, & Cicchetti (1984)	0;0–18;11	Receptive communication (includes items addressing pragmatics, semantics, syntax, morphology, and phonology)
			Expressive communication (includes items addressing pragmatics, semantics, syntax, morphology, and phonology)

mance on particular test items, and not develop intervention goals that are designed to teach test items.

Clinicians can gain impressions of underlying psycholinguistic functions by observing children's behaviors during testing. A number of behaviors we look for during testing are listed in Table 3.6.

Summary

We have proposed a framework for language assessment that enables clinicians to collect the data they need to determine whether children present temporary or permanent deviations from generally accepted standards of language knowledge and use. This determination requires careful consideration of language functions, language activities that children engage in, and the level of their participation in their daily activities. When clinicians interview parents, teachers, and children; when they collect language samples; when they perform dynamic assessments; when they review portfolios; when they observe children in natural settings; and when they augment this information with data from contextual and decontextual measures, they will be in the best position possible to determine whether children present language impairments.

TABLE 3.6 Observation of children's behavior during testing

Persistence
    Attempts to distract examiner from testing
    Attempts to answer before questions are completed
    Inappropriate responses to test items
    Complains about tasks
    Expresses concern over test performance
    Makes excuses for task failures
    Blames others for failures
Attentiveness
    Listens to directions
    Answers when queried or prompted
    Willingly accepts examiner assistance or suggestions
    Completes work within required time limits
    Remains focused on the tasks at hand
    Responds positively to attempts to establish rapport
    Listens attentively before responding
    Does not give up easily
Inattentiveness
    Fidgety, difficulty sitting still
    Distracted by outside noises
    Distracted by objects or pictures in the room
Avoidance
    Unusually slow in responding to items
    Must be reminded to focus on tasks
    Requests frequent breaks
    Performance deteriorates toward end of testing
    Forgets directions
Cooperativeness
    Seeks examiner's approval
    Tries to assist examiner
    Makes strong effort to solve test items
    Responds well to limits imposed by the test situation
    Follows directions
Uncooperativeness
    Reluctant to attempt tasks
    Initiates unrelated conversation during testing

References

American Educational Research Association, American Psychological Association, and National Council on Measurement in Education (1985). *Standards for educational and psychological testing*. Washington, DC: American Psychological Association.

Carrow-Woolfolk, E. (1995). *Oral and written language scales*. Circle Pines, MN: American Guidance Service.

Cole, K. N., Mills, P. E., & Dale, P. S. (1989). Examination of test-retest and split-half reliability for measures derived from language samples of young handicapped children. *Language, Speech, and Hearing Services in the Schools, 20*, 259–268.

Dickson, T., Linder, T. W., & Hudson, P. (1997). Observation of communication and language development. In T. W. Linder (Ed.), *Transdisciplinary play-based assessment* (pp. 163–215). Baltimore, MD: Brookes.

Dollaghan, C. A., & Campbell, T. F. (1992). A procedure for classifying disruptions in spontaneous language samples. *Topics in Language Disorders, 12*, 56–68.

Dunn, M., Rax, J., Sliwinski, M., & Aram, D. (1996). The use of spontaneous language measures as criteria for identifying children with specific language impairment: An attempt to reconcile clinical and research incongruence. *Journal of Speech and Hearing Research, 39*, 643–654.

Evans, J. L. (1996). Plotting the complexities of language sample analysis: Linear and nonlinear dynamical models of assessment. In K. N. Cole (Ed.), *Assessment of communication and language, Vol. 6: Communication and language intervention series* (pp. 207–256). Baltimore, MD: Brookes.

Evans, J. L., & Craig, H. K. (1992). Language sample collection and analysis: Interview compared to freeplay assessment contexts. *Journal of Speech and Hearing Research, 35*, 343–353.

Fey, M. E. (1988). *Language intervention with young children*. San Diego: College-Hill.

Gillam, R. B. (1990). An investigation of the oral language, reading, and written language competencies of language-learning impaired and normally achieving school-age children. *Dissertation Abstracts International, 50*, 3918.

Gillam, R. B., & Carlile, R. M. (1997). Oral reading and story retelling of students with specific language impairment. *Language, Speech, and Hearing Services in the Schools, 28*, 30–42.

Gillam, R. B., Peña, E. D., & Miller, L. (1999). Dynamic assessment of narrative and expository discourse. *Topics in Language Disorders, 20*, 33–47.

Goodman, Y. M., Watson, D. J., & Burke, C. L. (1987). *Reading miscue inventory: Alternative procedures*. New York: Richard C. Owen.

Hadley, P. A. (1998). Language sampling protocols for eliciting text-level discourse. *Language, Speech, and Hearing Services in Schools, 29*, 132–147.

Hammill, D. D. (1998). *Detroit tests of learning aptitude* (4th ed.). Austin, TX: Pro-ed.

Hammill, D., Brown, J., Larsen, S., & Weiderholt, LJ. (1994). *Test of adolescent and adult language*. Austin, TX: Pro-Ed.

Hunt, K. W. (1965). *Grammatical structures written at three grade levels*. Urbana, IL: National Council of Teachers of English.

Kemp, K., & Klee, T. (1997). Clinical language sampling practices: Results of a survey of speech-language pathologists in the United States. *Child Language Teaching and Therapy, 13,* 161–176.

Leadholm, B., & Miller, J. (1992). *Language sample analysis: The Wisconsin guide*. Madison, WI: Wisconsin Department of Public Instruction.

McCauley, R. J., & Swisher, L. (1984). Use and misuse of norm-referenced tests in clinical assessment: A hypothetical case. *Journal of Speech and Hearing Disorders, 49,* 338–348.

Miller, J. F., & Chapman, R. S. (1998). *Systematic analysis of language transcripts*. Madison, WI: Language Analysis Laboratory, Waisman Research Center.

Miller, L., Gillam, R., & Peña, E. (2000). *Dynamic assessment and intervention of children's narratives*. Austin, TX: Pro-Ed.

Miller, L. S. (2000a). *Two Friends*. Austin, TX: Neon Rose.

Miller, L. S. (2000b). *Bird and His Ring*. Austin, TX: Neon Rose.

Newcomer, P. L., & Hammill, D. D. (1997). *Test of language development—primary* (3rd ed.). Austin, TX: Pro-Ed.

Patterson, S., & Gillam, R. B. (1995). Team collaboration in the evaluation of language in students above the primary grades. In D. Tibbits (Ed.), *Language intervention: Beyond the primary grades* (pp. 137–181). Austin, TX: Pro-Ed.

Peña, E. D., & Gillam, R. B. (2000). Dynamic assessment of children referred for speech and language evaluations. In C. S. Lidz (Ed.), *Dynamic assessment: Prevailing models and applications*. Greenwich, CT: JAI.

Semel, E., Wiig, E., & Secord, W. (1996). *Clinical evaluation of language fundamentals* (3rd ed.). San Antonio, TX: Psychological Corporation.

Silliman, E. R., & Wilkinson, L. C. (1994). Observation is more than looking. In G. P. Wallach & K. G. Butler (Eds.), *Language learning disabilities in school-age children and adolescents: Some principles and applications* (pp. 145–173). New York: Merrill.

Sparrow, S., Balla, D., & Cicchetti, D. (1984). *Vineland adaptive behavior scales*. Circle Pines, MN: American Guidance Service.

Stockman, I. J. (1996). The promises and pitfalls of language sample analysis as an assessment tool for linguistic minority children. *Language, Speech, and Hearing Services in Schools, 27,* 355–366.

Tallal, P., Allard, L., Miller, S., & Curtiss, S. (1997). Academic outcomes of language impaired children. In C. Hulme & M. Snowling (Eds.), *Dyslexia: Biology, cognition, and intervention* (pp. 166–181). London: Whurr Publishers.

Tomblin, J. B., Records, N. L., & Zhang, X. (1996). A system for the diagnosis of specific language impairment in kindergarten children. *Journal of Speech and Hearing Research, 39,* 1284–1294.

Wagner, R. K., Torgesen, J. K., & Rashotte, C. A. (1999). *Comprehensive test of phonological processing*. Austin, TX: Pro-Ed.

Westby, C. E. (1990). Ethnographic interviewing: Asking the right questions to the right people in the right ways. *Journal of Childhood Communication Disorders, 13,* 101–111.

Wetherby, A. M., & Prizant, B. M. (1992). Facilitating language and communication development in autism: Assessment and intervention guidelines. In E. B. Dianne (Ed.), *Autism: Identification, education, and treatment* (pp. 107–134). Hillsdale, NJ: Lawrence Erlbaum.

Wiig, E., Secord, W., & Semel, E. (1992). *Clinical evaluation of language fundamentals* (3rd ed). San Antonio, TX: Psychological Corporation.

World Health Organization (1999—Beta-2 Draft. Full version ed. 1999). *ICIDH-2: International classification of functioning and disability.* Geneva: Author.

Zimmerman, I., Steiner, V., & Pond, R. (1992). *Preschool language scale—3.* San Antonio, TX: Psychological Corporation.

APPENDIX 3.A   Initial Parent Interview*

Explain who you are and why you are calling. For example:

Mrs. Jones, I'm Ron Gillam, and I'm the speech and language specialist at Michael's school. As you know, Michael's teacher has referred him for testing to determine whether he has speech, language, or learning difficulties. I'm calling you today because I'd like to understand Michael's communication abilities better before I see him.

First, what is the most important thing I should know about Michael? Is there anything about Michael's medical history that I should know about?

Psychological functions (competence)

1. What does Michael do really well?
    Listen for information about intellectual skills (attention, perception, memory, reasoning) and communication skills (speech production, language comprehension, and language production).

2. Is there anything Michael has difficulty doing?
    Listen for information about intellectual skills (attention, perception, memory, reasoning) and communication skills (speech production, language comprehension, and language production). Ask follow-up questions as necessary.
    a. Has he had trouble with this for a long time?
        Listen for developmental and medical information that would help you understand this problem better.
    b. Has anyone else ever noticed this besides you?
        Answers to this question may give you some insight into social/cultural expectations or environmental factors that support or hinder the child's abilities.
    c. What have you or someone else done to help Michael with this difficulty?
        Listen for information about support from family, friends, caregivers, teachers, or other members of their community.

3. Think about times when Michael has learned something new, like a new word or a new way of doing something (such as riding a bike, or playing a game).
    a. How would you describe Michael as a learner?
    b. How easily does Michael learn new things?
    c. How well does Michael pay attention when you are trying to teach him something?
    d. How well does Michael remember what you tell him?
    e. How well does Michael solve problems?

4. How would you compare Michael's ability to communicate with other children his age?
    a. How well do people understand Michael when he talks?
    b. How well does Michael understand what other people say?

c.   Have you ever noticed a difference between your ability to understand Michael and other's people's ability to understand him?

d.   How well does Michael explain himself?

Communication activities and level of involvement

5.   Would you please describe a typical day for Michael, from the time he gets up to the time he goes to bed?

Listen for clues about communication activities the child is involved in, the child's level of participation, and environmental supports or hindrances. Follow up this question with open-ended questions to obtain more details about parent perceptions of basic communication abilities, the activities the child is involved in, the level of participation in these activities, and environmental factors that support or hinder the child's involvement.

As you continue on from this point, remember that some of the questions may not be necessary after your initial follow-up questions.

6.   Who does Michael talk to routinely?

Listen for information about relatives, friends, teachers, caregivers.

7.   What does Michael like to talk about?

8.   When Michael talks to you, does he tell you things even before you ask?

a.   Does Michael ask you questions?

b.   Does he bring up new topics and ask questions when he is talking to friends, relatives, and teachers?

9.   Can you give me an example of the kinds of things Michael would be likely to say if he were telling you about something that happened while he was playing with a friend?

10. Does Michael take part in any organized recreational activities such as sports, boys' clubs, 4H, or after school care? If so, how much is he involved in these activities?

11. Does Michael take part in any religious activities? If so, how involved is he in these activities?

Environmental factors

12. Who encourages and supports Michael the most?

13. What kinds of things do they encourage him to do?

14. Is there anyone or anything that hinders Michael's involvement in any of the activities you want him to engage in?

---

*Reprinted with permission from Ronald B. Gillam, Ph.D., Jesse H. Jones Communication Center, Austin, Texas. Copyright © 2000.

APPENDIX 3.B   Language Sampling Protocol for Collecting Conversation and Narrative Samples*

Conversation: 15 minutes in length

1. Play with clay
2. Activities from classroom units

Introduce at least one topic absent in time and space from the sampling condition:

1. Holidays—what did you do, what will you do?
2. Family activities, visits, locations, etc.
3. Family pets
4. How to play a favorite game

Questions and prompts to facilitate talk in conversational contexts:
The following questions and prompts have been used effectively in the past. Do not limit yourself to these examples—use whatever works for you.

Conversation: Clay
"I've bought some clay for us to play with today."
"I wonder what we could make together?"
Follow the child's suggestions; request directions; ask "I'm going to make ____. What do I need to do it?"; or comment on the child's activity with the clay.

Conversation: Classroom activities, etc.
"Tell me about some of the things you've been doing in school lately." Ask about specific classroom units. "Did you do anything special for Halloween (etc.)? Tell me about that."
"Are you going to do anything special for Christmas?"
"Are you going to visit your grandma, grandpa?" "Where do they live?"
"How do you get there?" "What do you do there?"
"Do you have any pets at home?" "Tell me about them." "What do you have to do to take care of them?"

Narration: 15 minutes in length

1. Tell a favorite story.
2. Retell an episode from a TV program.
3. Retell a familiar story: "Goldilocks and the Three Bears," "Little Red Riding Hood," or "The Three Little Pigs." Picture prompts may be used only after every attempt has been made to elicit spontaneous speech.

Questions and prompts to facilitate talk in narrative contexts:

Narration TV
"Do you watch TV?"
"What programs do you like?"

"Tell me about that one, I haven't seen it."

"What happened on the last one you watched?"

"Do you ever watch (insert current program likely to be of interest)?"

Narration story

"Do you know any stories?"

"What is one of your favorite stories?"

"Oh, I don't know that one very well, will you tell it?"

"Do you know 'Little Red Riding Hood', etc.?" "Ooo, tell me about that one."

Use prompts as necessary, but make them open ended: "Can you tell me more?" "What else happened?"

You can use picture books for the familiar stories for the 3-year-olds, if necessary. Have books for the stories you think the children will know.

---

*Reprinted with permission from Leadholm, B., & Miller J. (1992). *Language sample analysis: The Wisconsin guide* (pp. 20–21). Madison, WI: Wisconsin Department of Public Instruction.

APPENDIX 3.C A Step-By-Step Language Analysis Procedure*

1. Transcribe the sample. Include all child and adult utterances. Mark unintelligible words as xx. Follow *Language Sample Analysis* (Lead-holm & Miller, 1992) transcription conventions.
2. Note mazes within parentheses ( ).
3. Place a / between all grammatical morphemes.
4. Decide whether each utterance is grammatically acceptable or unacceptable (take the child's dialect into consideration).
5. Decide how many clauses are contained in the sentence. Is it a phrase, a simple sentence, or a complex sentence?
6. Count the total number of words and the total number of different words, excluding words in mazes.
7. Decide whether each utterance is assertive or responsive (Fey, 1988).

Assertive utterances	Responsive utterances
Requests	Responses to questions
Descriptions/explanations	Acknowledgments
Comments	Imitations

8. Scan the sample for difficulties with form, content, or use. Describe each form, content, or use error.

Examples of common types of errors:

Content	Form	Use
Incorrectly used words	Word/morpheme omissions	Poor topic maintenance
Word retrieval problems	Word order errors	Poor turn taking
Inappropriate pronouns	Subject-verb agreement errors	Does not acknowledge speaker's message
Lack of coherence	Tense errors	Tangential comments
Nonspecific referents	Conjunction errors	Unstated referents

9. Calculate MLU and TTR. Use the LSA to determine MLU *z* score.
10. Make a distribution table for utterance length. Chart number of utterances as a function of utterance length in morphemes.

2	3	4	5	6	7	8

11. Make an acceptability/complexity table. Note the percentage of utterances that fall into each category.

	Grammatically acceptable	Grammatically unacceptable
Phrase		
Simple sentence		
Complex sentence		

12. Make an error chart. Note the percentage of utterances that contain the following kinds of errors.

Content	Form	Use

13. Summarize your results.

APPENDIX 3.D   Rules for Segmenting Utterances into C-Units*

There are two steps in transcribing stories into C-units.

Rule 1: Discover the boundaries. Listen for pauses and sentence ending intonation (rising pitch on questions or falling pitch on statements). A C-unit can be an incomplete utterance. This sometimes happens when children create dialog in their stories. For example:

The dog asked him, "Where's the cat?"

"Over there."

"Oh, okay."

Then they saw some fish.

Rule 2: Segment utterances before a new main clause or a coordinated clause. Children sometimes chain many clauses together, or they talk very quickly with fleeting pauses. When this happens, the C-unit consists of the main clause and all subordinate clauses that are attached to it.

The main clause consists of the subject, the main verb, and objects of the main verb, which combine to express the main idea in a sentence. For example, "My cat jumped on him" and "He was yelling" are single C-units that each have one main clause.

There is a simple rule to follow when clauses are conjoined by coordinating conjunctions (and, but, or so). If a subject is stated or restated after the coordinating conjunction (John was yelling, and Susan was laughing at him.), segment the utterance just before the conjunction (John was yelling. And Susan was laughing at him.). If no subject is stated after the coordinating conjunction, do not segment the utterances until the next main clause appears (e.g., John was running and yelling at the same time.).

A C-unit can contain any number of subordinating (dependent) clauses. Here are some examples:

- Subordinating conjunction: My cat jumped on her *because* she wanted to.
- Adverbial clause: My cat jumped on her *right after she came in*.
- Complement: She thought, *I don't even like cats*.
- Dialogue complement: She said, "*Get your cat off me*."
- Relative clause: The cat *that my brother found* jumped on my friend's lap.
- Infinitives: My cat likes *to jump* on people's laps.

One caution to keep in mind is that "so" can be a coordinating conjunction or a subordinating conjunction. If adding the word "that" after "so" fits grammatically into children's sentences, "so" is a subordinating conjunction; if not, "so" is a coordinating conjunction. For example:

- Coordinating conjunction (2 C-units): My cat jumped on her. So she got mad.
- Subordinating conjunction (1 C-unit): I held my cat so she wouldn't jump on my friend.

---

*Reprinted with permission from Ronald B. Gillam, Ph.D., Jesse H. Jones Communication Center, Austin, Texas. Copyright © 2000.

APPENDIX 3.E   Checklist of Behaviors to Watch for When Observing Young Children in Their Natural Environments*

Observation Guidelines for Communication and Language Development

I. Modalities of communication
   A. What is the primary method of communication used by the child?
      1. Eye gaze
      2. Gesture
      3. Physical manipulation
      4. Vocalization (nonspeech, e.g., grunts)
      5. Sign language
         a. Idiosyncratic
         b. Formal
      6. Verbalization
      7. Augmentation (e.g., symbol board)
   B. What supplemental forms are used in communication?
   C. What is the frequency of communication acts?
II. Pragmatics
   A. What pragmatic stage or level of intention is demonstrated by the child?
      1. Perlocutionary stage (lack of specific intent is demonstrated by the child)
      2. Illocutionary stage (use conventional gestures or vocalizations to communicate intentions)
      3. Locutionary stage (use of words to show intent)
   B. What meaning is implied by the child's gestures, vocalizations, and verbalizations?
      1. Seeking attention
      2. Requesting object
      3. Requesting action
      4. Requesting information
      5. Protesting
      6. Commenting on an object
      7. Greeting
      8. Answering
      9. Acknowledging other's speech
      10. Other
   C. What functions does the child's communication fulfill?
      1. Instrumental (to satisfy needs or desires)
      2. Regulatory (to control the behavior of others)
      3. Interactional (to define or participate in social interchange)
      4. Personal (to express opinions or feelings)
      5. Imaginative (to engage in fantasy)
      6. Heuristic (to obtain information)
      7. Informative (to provide information)
   D. What discourse skills does the child demonstrate (typically or optimally)?
      1. Attend to speaker
      2. Initiating conversation

        3. Turn-taking
        4. Maintaining a topic
        5. Volunteering/changing a topic
        6. Responding to requests for clarification
        7. Questioning
    E. Does the child demonstrate echolalia in communication?
        1. Timing
            a. Immediate
            b. Delayed
        2. Echolalia
            a. Exact
            b. Mitigated
        3. Function
            a. To continue interaction
            b. To demonstrate comprehension
        4. Degree of pragmatic success
III. Phonology: Sound production patterns
    A. What phonemes or speech sounds are produced by the child?
        1. Preverbal sounds
        2. Speech sounds
        3. Babbling–consonant–vowel combinations
        4. Jargon—speech sounds combined into patterns with cultural intonations
        5. Words
    B. Phonological processes or errors
        1. Deletions
            a. Consonants
            b. Syllables
            c. Sounds
        2. Assimilations (one sound becomes similar to another in the same word)
        3. Substitutions
            a. Initial sounds
            b. Final sounds
            c. For liquids, /l/ and /r/
            d. Vowels
    C. Intelligibility level (percentage of verbalizations understood)
        1. In known context
        2. In unknown context
        3. By familiar person or family member
        4. Appropriateness of intonation
        5. Dysfluencies or stuttering
IV. Semantic and syntactic understanding
    A. What cognitive level of understanding is demonstrated in the child's language?
        1. Referential (specific objects)
        2. Extended (more than one object)

3. Relational (relations between objects)
4. Categorical (discrimination and classification)
5. Metalinguistic (talking about language)

B. What types of words are used?
   1. Nouns
   2. Verbs
   3. Adjectives
   4. Adverbs
   5. Prepositions
   6. Negatives
   7. Conjunctions

C. What semantic relations are expressed in the child's language?
   1. Agent (*baby*)
   2. Action (*drink*)
   3. Object (*cup*)
   4. Recurrence (*more*)
   5. Nonexistence (*all gone*)
   6. Cessation (*stop*)
   7. Rejection (*no*)
   8. Location (*up*)
   9. Possession (*mine*)
   10. Agent-action (*baby drink*)
   11. Action-object (*drink juice*)
   12. Agent–action–object (*baby drink juice*)
   13. Action–object–location (*throw ball up*)
   14. Other

D. What type of sentences are used by the child?
   1. Structure
      a. Declarative
      b. Imperative
      c. Negative
      d. Questions
   2. Level of complexity
      a. Simple
      b. Compound
      c. Complex

E. What morphological markers does the child use?
   1. Present progressive (*-ing*)
   2. Prepositions (*in, on*)
   3. Regular and irregular past tense (*-ed, came*)
   4. Possessives (*'s*)
   5. Contractible and uncontractible copula (*dog's little, he is,* in response to question, "*Who is happy?*")
   6. Regular and irregular third person (*jumps, does*)
   7. Contractible and uncontractible auxiliary (*Mommy's drinking, he is,* in response to question, "*Who is combing his hair?*")

F. What is the child's mean length of utterance?

V. Comprehension of language
   A. What early comprehension is demonstrated?
      1. What is the child's reaction to sounds?
      2. Does the child exhibit joint referencing with an adult?
         a. With visual regard
         b. With verbal cue
         c. With physical cue
      3. Does the child respond to common routines or statements?
         a. With contextual cues
         b. Without contextual cues
   B. What comprehension of language forms is demonstrated?
      1. To which semantic relations does a child respond?
      2. To which questions does the child respond?
         a. Yes/no questions
         b. Simple "wh" questions (*where, what, who*)
         c. Advanced "wh" questions (*which, when, why, how*)
      3. What commands can the child follow?
         a. Complexity (one-step, multistep)
         b. With/without contextual cues
      4. What prepositions can the child understand?
         a. Simple (*in, on*)
         b. Advanced (*next to, behind, in front of*)
      5. What temporal terms does the child understand?
      6. What relational terms does the child understand?
VI. Oral motor development
   A. What cup drinking skills does the child demonstrate?
      1. Is the head aligned with the body?
         a. Midline
         b. Head extension or retraction
      2. What degree of lip control is seen?
         a. Degree of lip seal when cup to lips
         b. Ease with which jaw and lips meet cup
         c. Lip control when cup removed from mouth
      3. What degree of tongue control is seen?
         a. Degree of tongue protrusion under cup
         b. Lack of tongue thrust forward
      4. How does the child coordinate suck/swallow?
         a. Sequence of suck/swallow
         b. Amount child can drink without pause
         c. Can inhibit breathing while swallowing
         d. Frequency of coughing and choking
   B. How adept is the child at chewing and swallowing solids?
      1. Can the child sustain and control bite?
      2. What jaw movement is observed?
         a. Bite release
         b. Rotary pattern—diagonal
         c. Rotary pattern—circular

    3.   To what degree does the tongue assist in moving food from side to side?

    4.   What degree of lip control is seen?
       a.   Movement is independent of jaw
       b.   Mouth closure
       c.   Amount of food loss or salivation while chewing

VII. Observations related to other areas

  A. Hearing

  B. Voice quality

  C. Cognitive development
    1.   What level of imitations is indicated in the child's language?
       a.   Motor acts
       b.   Oral motor acts
       c.   Speech and nonspeech sounds
       d.   Word approximations
       e.   Words (one-syllable, two-syllable, multisyllable)
       f.   Word combinations (two-word, three-word, etc.)
       g.   Complete sentences
       h.   Morphologic markers

    2.   What cognitive prerequisites to language are evident?
       a.   Object permanence (ability to represent objects and events not perceptually present)
       b.   Means-end behaviors (actions to achieve a goal)
       c.   Functional object use and object classification (perception and relationships)
       d.   Symbolic behavior (ability to internalize and reproduce information)

  D. Social-emotional development
    1.   See pragmatic skills related to social interaction (see Chapter 6)
    2.   Are topics of communication appropriate?
    3.   Does the child communicate in a similar manner with all partners?

  E. Sensorimotor development
    1.   Visual-motor skills
    2.   Muscle tone and postural control
    3.   Reflexes
    4.   Fine motor skills
    5.   Motor planning

---

*Reprinted with permission from T. W. Linder. (1997). Observation guidelines for communication and language development. In T. W. Linder (Ed.), *Transdisciplinary play-based assessment* (pp. 179–186). Baltimore, MD: Brookes.

CLASSROOM LANGUAGE OBSERVATION

Student: _____ Teacher: _____ Date: _____

Observer: _____ Position: _____

COMMUNICATION ACTS	STUDENT	PEER
Assertive Acts		
Requests (utterances that solicit information or actions)		
Comments (utterances that label, report facts, state rules, or state explanations)		
Responsive Acts		
Responses (utterances that provide information that has been requested)		
Acknowledgments (utterances that acknowledge but add no new information to prior utterances)		
Imitations (utterances that include all or part of prior utterances, including self-repetitions)		

Time:　　　　　　　　　 Begin____ End____ Begin____ End____

Discourse Level: I = Initiate Topic, M = Maintain Topic, E = Extend Topic

Content-Form Acceptability: Ⓘ Ⓜ Ⓔ = Syntactically unacceptable

 + M E = Semantically unacceptable

Context: _____

_____

Participants: _____

Comments: _____

_____

TOTALS:	Student	Peer			Student	Peer
# of Utterances						
# of Assertive Acts			% Assertive Acts			
# of Responsive Acts			% Responsive Acts			
# of Initiating			% Initiating			
# of Maintaining			% Maintaining			
# of Extending			% Extending			
# of Synt. Unacc.			% Synt. Unacc.			
# of Semant. Unacc.			% Semant. Unacc.			

*Reprinted with permission from Patterson, S., & Gillam, R. B. (1995). Team collaboration in the evaluation of language in students above the primary grades. In D. Tibbits (Ed.), *Language intervention: Beyond the primary grades* (pp. 137–181). Austin, TX: Pro-Ed (pp. 161 and 163).

APPENDIX 3.G Examining Portfolios and Homework Assignments*

Questions to consider include:

1. What instructions were given to the child?
   a. Were they oral or written?
   b. Examine the level of complexity and redundancy.
2. Was the child expected to work independently or with others?
   a. To what degree did the child follow through on this? Why or why not?
3. What questions did the child ask while completing the task?
   a. To whom, when, and how?
4. What support resources were available to the child while completing the task (persons, objects, etc.)?
   a. Did the child attempt to use these? How?
   b. Were these attempts successful?
5. What is the overall quality of the product?
6. How does the product compare with that of his or her peers?
7. How do products within the same content area (language arts, mathematics, social studies, art) compare across time?
   a. Is there variability present?
   b. Is variability consistent with developing skills?
   c. Are there other factors that may contribute to variability of performance, such as type of activity, topic, persons present?
8. What syntactic/semantic errors are evident within the products?
9. How do the products compare with spoken language?
10. Was there a time limit to the task? How did this appear to influence the child's performance?
11. In what ways is the product similar to the child's peers? Different? Which aspects of the product could the child produce independently? With a little assistance? With moderate assistance? Not at all? What evidence is present for the child's strengths?
14. How does the teacher regard the child's products?
15. How do the parents regard the child's products?
16. How does the child regard his or her own products?

---

*Reprinted with permission from Ronald B. Gillam, Ph.D., Jesse H. Jones Communication Center, Austin, Texas. Copyright © 1999.

APPENDIX 3.H Marking Reading Miscue Inventory Transcripts*

Substitutions: Write the participant's miscue directly above the author-intended word:

> *cloth*
> James put a sheet over the table.

Omissions: Words that are omitted during reading are circled:

> Ginger asked, "(How) could you tell?"

Insertions: Words that are added to the text are marked by placing a caret (^) between the text items where the insertion occurred and by writing the reader's miscue above the caret:

> *about*
> When the tiger heard ^ this, he was so frightened that he bounded into the forest.

Repetitions of words or phrases: The portion of the text that is repeated is underlined, with the left end of the line forming a circle around the letter "R":

> ®
> James showed Ginger⌐how to do the trick.

Corrections of words or phrases: Repetitions in which the reader corrected his or her miscue are marked similarly, except with an encircled "C" to the left of the underlined text:

> ©*kept*
> "And I⌐keep warm by fluttering my wings," said the hummingbird.

(In the example above, the student read, "'And I kept . . . keep warm by fluttering my wings,' said the hummingbird.")

Abandoning a correct word or phrase: When readers regress and abandon a correct production, the repeated portion of the text is underlined. The letters "AC" (abandon correct) are encircled to the left of the underlined text:

> (AC) *light*
> Another would walk in front of him with the⌐lighted lantern to show him the way.

(In this case the reader read, "Another would walk in front of him with the lighted . . . light lantern to show him the way.")

---

*Reprinted with permission from Ronald B. Gillam, Ph.D. Jesse J. Jones Communication Center, Austin, Texas. Copyright © 2000.

4   Aphasia Testing

Carl A. Coelho
Mary Boyle

Assessment has been described as the process of gathering data about the impairment (the underlying neurologic disorder), the disability (the decreased functional communicative ability resulting from the impairment), and the handicap (the decreased ability of the individual to communicate in the context of expected social roles). Decisions about the clinical course of action are made on the basis of that information. Treatment planning, therefore, may be viewed as the outcome of the assessment process (Yorkston et al., 1988).

With regard to the assessment of aphasia, Linebaugh (1979) has noted that information obtained from a test of aphasia may be used for a variety of general purposes:

1.   Differential diagnosis
2.   Localization of lesion
3.   Determination of patient's level of functional communication
4.   Establishment of a prognosis
5.   Focusing treatment
6.   Assessment of recovery and effectiveness of treatment

Each of these six general purposes is discussed in this chapter.

Differential Diagnosis

The first task in the assessment process with a neurologic communication disorder is to make a series of differentiations:

- Are the individual's communication skills impaired or within normal limits?
- If communication is impaired, is it language specific (i.e., aphasia) or a reflection of some other primary disturbance (e.g., TBI or dementia)?

- Is the impairment limited to only language processes (i.e., morphology, phonology, and syntax), or does it involve motor planning and programming or execution for speech (i.e., apraxia of speech or dysarthria)?

These differentiations are critical not only for their contribution to the medical diagnosis, but for their implications in determining the patient's candidacy for therapy and the nature of therapy.

A number of factors contribute to the differential diagnosis process. Included are

- Fluency with which a patient produces speech (the assessment protocol should provide for the elicitation of verbal responses encompassing a wide range of length and complexity)
- Degree of impairment of specific communicative abilities (to provide adequate data for differentiating among various aphasic and non-aphasic communication impairments, the assessment protocol should include tasks in all language modalities covering a wide range of difficulty)
- Patient's response patterns on nonlanguage tasks (such nonlanguage tasks are included to assess specific processes that subserve language— for example, attention and memory, the integrity of which are necessary prerequisites to successful performance on speech and language tasks)
- Type of responses produced by the patient (if we are to fully understand the nature of a patient's communication impairment, a detailed analysis of his or her responses is required in which we then seek to infer the mediating processes by which they were produced)
- Relevance of the patient's responses to test stimuli (errors of relevance involve bizarre responses that appear unrelated to the stimulus)
- Awareness of errors and the ability to self-correct

Localization

Particular patterns of speech and language impairment may be related to involvement of specific regions of the central nervous system. The development of increasingly sophisticated neuroradiologic procedures (e.g., computed tomography scans, magnetic resonance imaging, positron emission tomography scans, etc.) has minimized the need for making an inferential leap between behaviors and specific brain regions. However, careful description of an individual's speech and language impairment and delineation of error patterns significantly contribute to the overall process of reaching or confirming a neurologic diagnosis.

Determining Level of Functional Communication

Attempts at determining patients' performance in natural communicative situations may involve predicting such performance from scores on standardized tasks used in formal testing. An example of this would be to use the Aphasia Severity Rating Scale from the Boston Diagnostic Aphasia Examination (BDAE; Goodglass & Kaplan, 1972); in particular, the portion of the communicative burden carried by the listener. A second, more direct strategy is to assess performance in tasks approaching natural communication situations. An example of this would be to use the Communicative Abilities in Daily Living (CADL; Holland et al., 1999) or to use rating scales, such as the Functional Communication Profile (Sarno, 1969) or the Communicative Effectiveness Index (Lomas et al., 1989), in which functional communication is rated by the clinician or other care providers. A third approach to the determination of functional performance is through the use of any of a variety of functional status measures that are being used by most rehabilitation centers to determine outcomes of extended rehabilitation for neurologic patients. Such measures include the Functional Independence Measure (State University of New York at Buffalo, 1990), the Patient Evaluation and Conference System (Harvey & Jellinek, 1979), the Rancho Rehabilitation Outcome Evaluation (Rancho Los Amigos Medical Center, 1993), and the Rehabilitation Institute of Chicago—Functional Assessment Scales (Heinemann, 1993), in which communication skills are one dimension of a patient's "functional status" that is rated. A major limitation of all of these data management systems used for measuring rehabilitation outcomes is that they are not sophisticated or sensitive enough to detect small increments of functional change, particularly in the area of communication skills. In response to speech-language pathologists' concern with these functional outcome scales, the Functional Assessment of Communication Skills for Adults measure was developed and validated with both head-injured and aphasic inpatients (Frattali et al., 1995). Preliminary findings have indicated that this measure is sensitive to improvement in functional outcome during inpatient speech-language intervention.

Establishment of a Prognosis

Perhaps one of the most challenging clinical endeavors is predicting the eventual extent of an individual's recovery. Patient variables such as age, time postonset, and site and extent of lesion are considered to be predictive in certain neurologic conditions. Length of coma, initial degree of impairment in auditory comprehension, overall severity of communicative impairment, and severity of left neglect are thought to be predictive in others.

Focusing Treatment

The most important use of the information derived from speech and language testing is that it be reliably used for focusing treatment. Whether it be a list of psycholinguistic or information processing factors for an aphasic patient, or an analysis of components of normal speech production for a dysarthric patient, this assessment protocol should yield the level of breakdown (i.e., that point at which the patient begins to experience difficulty) or identify the component that, if addressed in therapy, might achieve the greatest impact on communication function.

Assessing Recovery and Effectiveness of Treatment

For performance to be compared across time (i.e., pre- to post-treatment), some form of standard score must be used (e.g., aphasia quotient from the Western Aphasia Battery [WAB; Kertesz, 1982] or overall score from the Porch Index of Communicative Ability [PICA; Porch, 1981a], which uses a sensitive scoring system that reflects subtle changes in the patients' performance and has a high degree of test stability over time). Whenever possible, traditional assessment procedures should be supplemented by functional assessment techniques. Such procedures include observation, questionnaires, checklists, and rating scales. Functional assessment determines current level of functioning and assists in the determination of optimal approaches to intervention. Giles (1994) notes that functional assessment is central to the selection of goals and target behaviors required for the rehabilitation team's integrated treatment plan. Functional assessments should be conducted under conditions as close as possible to those the individual will experience after rehabilitation. The rigorous control of extraneous variables necessary for standardized assessments is sacrificed in favor of ecologic validity. There are many variables that may influence performance in real world situations, such as setting (where the individual is at a particular point in time), cues (events that facilitate the production of a behavior), or environmental conditions (who else is present, level of activity, time of day, etc.). Patient observation enables clinicians to identify skills that appear to be intact or functional in the sterile clinical setting but are actually nonfunctional in a home or work environment (Starch & Falltrick, 1990).

Specific Assessment Tools for Aphasia

In the following sections, a variety of tests of aphasia are described. Many of the observations about these aphasia tests are reflections of the authors' clinical experiences since the early 1980s. In most instances, assessment tools should be selected based on the diagnostic needs of a given aphasic individual as opposed to applying a given battery to all individuals. On certain occasions, selected subtests from more than one battery may be administered to the same individual to address special diagnostic concerns.

An important issue related to special diagnostic concerns involves the assessment of aphasic individuals from diverse cultural and linguistic backgrounds. In the ideal situation, such patients might be matched with clinicians who have attained bicultural and bilingual/bidialectal competency through specific academic and clinical training. When such matches cannot be made, the use of an interpreter may help to bridge the language and cultural gap between the patient and clinician. Wallace (1996) recommends the following general guidelines for monolingual clinicians called on to evaluate linguistically and culturally diverse patients:

- Obtain information about the individual's culture and language system.
- Become familiar with a few simple words in the individual's native language and be able to pronounce them correctly.
- Obtain information regarding nonverbal communication skills appropriate to the individual's culture and generation.
- Work with an interpreter throughout the assessment process.
- Select culturally and linguistically appropriate tasks to obtain comparable information across languages.
- Determine the most productive language with regard to assessment and treatment.

The aphasia tests reviewed here were selected because of their widespread clinical use in the United States. In addition, many of these tests have been subjected to empirical investigations. Four categories of assessment instruments are reviewed: comprehensive batteries, supplemental measures, tests for special purposes, and screening tools. For each test, a general description is provided along with normative information. The theoretical underpinnings and the clinical use of each test are also discussed.

Comprehensive Aphasia Batteries

In this section, four comprehensive aphasia batteries are discussed: the Minnesota Test for Differential Diagnosis of Aphasia (MTDDA), the BDAE, the WAB, and the PICA. These four tests are the most widely used aphasia batteries.

Minnesota Test for Differential Diagnosis of Aphasia
General Description
SUBTESTS
Subtests for the MTDDA include

- *Auditory disturbances*: Recognizing common words, discriminating between paired words, recognizing letters, identifying items named serially, understanding sentences, following directions, understanding a paragraph, repeating digits, repeating sentences
- *Visual and reading disturbances*: Matching forms, matching letters, matching words to pictures, matching printed to spoken words, reading comprehension—sentences, reading rate—sentences, reading comprehension—paragraphs, oral reading—words, oral reading—sentences
- *Speech and language disturbances*: Imitating gross movements, rapid alternating movements, repeating monosyllables, repeating phrases, counting to 20, naming days of the week, completing sentences, answering simple questions, giving biographic information,

expressing ideas, producing sentences, describing pictures, naming pictures, defining words, retelling paragraphs

- *Visuomotor and writing disturbances*: Copying Greek letters, writing numbers to 20, reproducing a wheel, reproducing letters, writing letters to dictation, written spelling, oral spelling, producing written sentences, writing sentences to dictation, writing a paragraph
- *Disturbances of numerical relations and arithmetic processes*: Making change, setting clock, simple numeric combinations, written problems

INTENT

The MTDDA was designed to determine the level at which aphasic language performance breaks down in each of the principal language modalities and to reveal the nature of the disruptions that occur.

TIME FOR ADMINISTRATION

The MTDDA is administered in 2–6 hours. To shorten testing time, it is recommended that a baseline (the test on which a patient makes only one error) and a ceiling (the test on which a patient fails 90% of the items) be obtained for each patient within each language modality, so that not all of the subtests need to be given. Shortened versions of the MTDDA have been proposed and studied (Powell et al., 1980; Thompson & Enderby, 1979).

SCORING

Most scoring is plus-minus, performed during test administration. A Diagnostic Scale and Clinical Ratings are completed after testing. The diagnostic scale indicates the nature and overall pattern of deficit that underlies the communication impairment and rates 12 specific behaviors on a 4-point scale from 0 (no impairment) to 3 (severe impairment). The clinical ratings estimate the severity level of impairment in five categories (understanding, speech, reading, writing, and dysarthria) on a 7-point scale (Table 4.1).

MATERIALS NEEDED FOR ADMINISTRATION

To administer the MTDDA, the following are needed:

1. Differential Diagnosis of Aphasia—Revised
2. *Administrative Manual for the Minnesota Test for Differential Diagnosis of Aphasia* (Schuell, 1965, 1972)
3. Test booklet
4. Card materials in two wirebound books

Normative Information (Standardization)

The test was developed and revised between 1948 and 1972 (Schuell, 1972). Statistical information (means, standard deviations, median scores, the percentage of subjects making errors on each subtest, factor analysis, and correlational data) published in *Differential Diagnosis of Aphasia—Revised* is based on subjects tested for the 1955 research edition and the 1965 published edition. Not all aphasic subjects were administered all of the subtests.

TABLE 4.1 Clinical rating (scale 0–6)

Understand what is said	Writing (underline hand: R, L; preferred, nonpreferred)
0 No observable impairment	0 No observable impairment
1 Follows radio program or general discussion with only minimal difficulty	1 Can write acceptable letter with only minimal errors
2 Follows ordinary conversation but sometimes fails to grasp essentials	2 Spontaneous writing present, with mild impairment of spelling and formulation
3 Follows most conversation but requires repetition	3 Can write short, essay sentences spontaneously and to dictation
4 Follows simple conversation but requires repetition	4 Spelling vocabulary of 100 or more words; can write some phrases and sentences
5 Follows brief statements with considerable repetition	5 Can write name and a few words to dictation
6 Usually responds inappropriately because does not understand	6 No functional writing

Speech	Dysarthria
0 No observable impairment	0 No observable impairment
1 Converse easily with occasional difficulty	1 Occasional hesitation or slurring
2 Conversational speech, with mild difficulty finding words or expressing ideas	2 Intelligible speech with mild slurring or slowness
3 Some conversational speech but marked difficulty in expressing long or complex ideas	3 Intelligible but obviously defective speech
4 Ready communication with single words and short phrases	4 Frequent omissions and substitutions of sounds
5 Expresses needs and wishes in limited or defective manner	5 Speech barely intelligible
6 No functional speech	6 Speech usually unintelligible

Reading

0 No observable impairment

1 Reads average adult materials with only minimal difficulty

2 Reads newspaper and short magazine materials

3 Reads simple sentences and simple paragraph materials

4 Reading vocabulary of 100 or more words, reads some phrases and sentences

5 Matches words to pictures and some spoken to printed words

6 No functional reading

Source: H. Schuell. *Booklet for the Minnesota Test for Differential Diagnosis of Aphasia*. Copyright © 1965, 1972 by the University of Minnesota. All rights reserved. Used by permission of the University of Minnesota Press.

POPULATIONS

The 1955 research edition included 157 aphasic subjects and 50 nonaphasic hospitalized subjects, and the 1965 published edition included 23 aphasic subjects. The aphasic subjects were described as neurologically stable with no evidence of psychosis or regressive behavior. In both the aphasic and nonaphasic groups, 38% of the subjects were younger than 50 years of age, and 62% were older than age 50. The aphasic subjects had a slightly higher educational and vocational level than the nonaphasic subjects.

INTERPRETATION OF SCORES

Schuell and her colleagues state that differential diagnosis isn't possible based on quantitative test scores alone, and that it is more meaningful to describe a patient's performance in terms of the kinds of errors made and the pattern of test performance.

PROFILES

The seven major categories of aphasia are described, with a definition, clinical signs, the most discriminating tests, and a prognosis provided for each category. The seven categories have been examined psychometrically (Powell et al., 1979) and are as follows:

1. Simple aphasia
2. Aphasia with visual involvement
3. Mild aphasia with persisting dysfluency
4. Aphasia with scattered findings
5. Aphasia with sensorimotor involvement
6. Aphasia with intermittent auditory imperception
7. Irreversible aphasic syndrome

Theoretical Biases of Authors

Schuell et al. (1965) argued that the difference between aphasic and non-aphasic disruption of language is largely quantitative rather than qualitative, so that there are different severity levels of aphasia, but not different kinds of aphasia. She defined aphasia as a *multimodal reduction of available language that may or may not be complicated by perceptual or sensorimotor involvement, by various forms of dysarthria, or by other sequelae of brain damage.* The overall pattern of involvement varies from patient to patient, making differential diagnosis possible. Schuell et al. (1965) felt that differential diagnosis serves as the basis of description, which guides treatment, and of prediction, which guides long-term planning.

Validity, Reliability, and Sensitivity

Construct validity was demonstrated through factor analysis (Schuell et al., 1962). Reliability was not assessed. Aphasic and nonaphasic subjects in the standardization samples were separable on the basis of magnitude and distribution of errors. Correlations between test sections were high for aphasic subjects and low for nonaphasic subjects.

Clinical Use

STRENGTHS

The MTDDA test allows for comprehensive evaluation of language behavior. Materials are well organized, portable, and easy to use.

The MTDDA requires a long administration time, even when the recommendations for shorter administration are followed.

WHAT IS THE TEST BEST SUITED FOR?
Judiciously selected subtests can probe specific aspects of language more deeply than most other aphasia batteries and therefore may serve as a useful adjunct to them. The clear, simple formatting of the picture cards may be useful with more severely impaired patients.

Boston Diagnostic Aphasia Examination
General Description
SUBTESTS
Subtests for the BDAE include

- *Conversational and expository speech*: responses to questions, open-ended conversation, picture description (using "cookie theft" picture)
- *Auditory comprehension*: word discrimination, body-part identification, commands, complex ideational material
- *Oral expression*: oral agility (nonverbal and verbal), automatized sequences, recitation, singing, rhythm, repetition of words, repeating phrases, word reading, responsive naming, visual confrontation naming, animal naming (fluency in controlled association), oral sentence reading
- *Understanding written language*: symbol and word discrimination, phonetic association (word recognition and comprehension of oral spelling), word-picture matching, reading sentences and paragraphs
- *Writing*: mechanics of writing, recall of written symbols (serial writing, primer-level dictation), written word-finding (spelling to dictation and written confrontation naming), written formulation

INTENT
The BDAE is designed to sample behaviors important for identification of aphasic syndromes. These behaviors include spontaneous connected verbalization and repetition. Diagnosis of a syndrome is accomplished by examining the pattern of results on the rating of speech characteristics and the subtest summary profile. The test manual provides examples and ranges of performance typically seen in cases of Broca's, Wernicke's, anomic, and conduction aphasias.

TIME FOR ADMINISTRATION
The BDAE is administered in 1–3 hours.

SCORING
Scoring varies among subtests: plus-minus scoring, 4-point scales, and frequency counts are used. Because possible scores vary from 8 or 10 points on some subtests to 105 points on confrontation naming, reporting of scores should be in terms of ratios.

MATERIALS NEEDED FOR ADMINISTRATION
To administer the BDAE, the following are needed:

1. *The Assessment of Aphasia and Related Disorders* (Goodglass & Kaplan, 1983a)
2. Sixteen stimulus cards
3. Scoring booklet

Normative Information (Standardization)

Some of the characteristic features of the BDAE first appeared in the literature in the early 1960s. For example, Goodglass et al. (1964) first described a rating profile of speech characteristics to distinguish features of aphasic spontaneous speech that later appeared in the BDAE. The test was first published in 1972 and revised in 1983 (Goodglass & Kaplan, 1983b).

POPULATIONS

The 1972 edition was normed on a sample of 207 aphasic patients. Demographic information (i.e., age, etiology, education, etc.) was not reported. A new set of norms was developed for the second edition. Performance on the BDAE by 147 normal adults taken from a study by Borod et al. (1980) is now reported in the manual. These data include means, standard deviations, and ranges for each subtest differentiated by age with performance reported by decade. Also included in the manual are normal scores for the spatial-quantitative battery distributed by age and education. A normative sample of 242 aphasic individuals replaces the sample reported in the first edition. It should be noted that this group was heavily loaded with individuals with focal lesions.

INTERPRETATION OF SCORES

Data from the second edition's normative group were used to relate raw scores to percentiles. Cutoff scores were derived from studies of normal adults. Lowest scores tended to be obtained by individuals older than 60 years of age with fewer than 9 years of education. Therefore, when assessing elderly patients, the cutoff scores should be relaxed before labeling their performance as disordered.

PROFILES

Aphasic syndromes are diagnosed through the examination of patterns of results on the rating of speech characteristics and the subtest summary profile. The BDAE manual provides examples and ranges of performance typically seen in patients with Broca's, Wernicke's, anomic, and conduction aphasias (e.g., see Appendices 4A and 4B).

Theoretical Biases of Authors

Goodglass and Kaplan believed the nature of an individual's aphasia was determined by the organization of language in the person's brain as well as the site of brain damage causing the aphasia. The BDAE, according to Goodglass and Kaplan, permits clinicians to determine the presence of aphasia and type of aphasia syndrome that leads to inferences related to cerebral localization (Goodglass & Kaplan, 1983b).

Validity, Reliability, and Sensitivity
The BDAE has been investigated as a measure of communicative ability by Holland (1980), who noted that the BDAE correlated at 0.84 with her CADL and at 0.49 with her criterion measure of real-world communication situations. Wertz et al. (1984) investigated the validity of the BDAE as to its classification of aphasias. Forty-five aphasic patients were given the BDAE and the WAB (Kertesz, 1982), also designed to identify aphasic syndromes. There was only 27% agreement as to classification of these patients. Naeser and Hayward (1978) have found agreement between independent classification with the BDAE and predicted site of damage determined with computed tomography scans for 19 subjects. Interexaminer reliability of the profile of speech characteristics has been reported to be 0.85 and higher. Correlations for identification of paraphasias and word-finding were somewhat lower—0.79 and 0.78, respectively.

Clinical Use
STRENGTHS
The BDAE provides a comprehensive assessment, sampling a broad array of language abilities. The profile of speech characteristics is a useful tool for characterizing spontaneous speech samples.

WEAKNESSES
The BDAE is not well suited for individuals with severe aphasia. Aphasic patients with larger nonfocal lesions may be difficult to categorize into aphasic syndromes.

WHAT IS THE TEST BEST SUITED FOR?
The BDAE is most appropriate for moderately impaired patients with aphasia secondary to focal lesions.

Western Aphasia Battery
General Description
SUBTESTS
Subtests for the WAB are grouped under seven main headings:

1. Spontaneous speech
2. Comprehension
3. Repetition
4. Naming
5. Reading and writing
6. Praxis
7. Construction

An *aphasia quotient*, an index of language impairment severity, is calculated using the subtests under the first five headings. A *cortical quotient*, which is an index of cognitive functions, is calculated using all of the subtests.

INTENT

This test was designed to evaluate language function and to assess non-verbal skills to obtain overall measures of severity and to allow classification of the aphasic patient according to aphasic syndrome.

TIME FOR ADMINISTRATION

According to the author (Kertesz, 1982), the oral portion of the test takes approximately an hour to administer to most patients, but it can be administered in individual sections on consecutive days. The reading, writing, calculation, and praxis subtests are considered as an independent unit, and these nonverbal tests are optional.

SCORING

Each item is scored as it is administered, with totals and subsequent calculations completed after the examination session. Scoring is fairly straightforward, with explicit instructions printed in the test booklet.

MATERIALS NEEDED FOR ADMINISTRATION

The following, all provided with the test package, are needed for administration of the WAB:

1. Test manual
2. Test booklet
3. Stimulus cards

In addition, 20 test objects must be obtained separately for use with the oral portion of the test. For the nonverbal tests, four Koh's blocks, and the Raven's Colored Progressive Matrices are required; these may be purchased from the same publisher. In addition, a stop-watch is needed, and 2-cm cardboard or wood letters must be cut out.

Normative Information (Standardization)

Initial normative data were obtained in 1974, with additional samples reported in 1979 and 1982. The only normative data reported in the manual are the correlation between the most recent (Kertesz, 1982) and previous (Kertesz, 1979) versions of the test. Normative information on the earlier version of the test is contained in papers by Kertesz (1979) and by Shewan and Kertesz (1980).

POPULATIONS

The 1974 sample used 150 aphasic subjects, 21 non–brain-injured subjects, and 17 subjects with unilateral hemispheric damage but no aphasia. In 1979, 215 aphasic subjects, 63 non–brain-injured subjects, and 53 non-aphasic brain-damaged subjects participated, and in 1982, results for 20 additional aphasic patients were reported. The samples included a variety of aphasic syndromes and etiologies.

INTERPRETATION OF SCORES

The aphasia quotient provides a measure of severity of language impairment, and performance greater than 93.8 on this measure is considered to be within normal limits. Subscores for fluency, comprehension, repetition, and naming are used to classify aphasic syndromes.

Criteria for classifying individuals into classical aphasia syndromes (global, Broca's, isolation, transcortical motor, Wernicke's, transcortical sensory, conduction, and anomic) are based on their subscores in fluency, comprehension, repetition, and naming.

Theoretical Biases of Authors

Kertesz (1982) supports a multidimensional theory of aphasia, which proposes that there are different syndromes of aphasia that reflect differential impairment in distinct components of the language system.

Validity, Reliability, and Sensitivity

Construct validity of the WAB's ability to classify patients has been questioned. Studies examining agreement between WAB and BDAE classification (Wertz et al., 1984) and agreement between WAB classification and clinician impression (Swindell et al., 1984) found agreement of only 27% and 54%, respectively. Some have criticized the WAB for forcing patients into diagnostic categories (Brookshire, 1997). Shewan and Kertesz (1980) reported strong test-retest reliability and strong interexaminer reliability for the WAB.

Clinical Use

STRENGTHS

The WAB provides an objective method of classifying aphasic patients based on subtest scores. It takes less time to administer than some other aphasia batteries, such as the PICA or the BDAE. Instructions for administration and scoring are straightforward.

WEAKNESSES

The WAB's objective classification system, considered a strength by some, has been criticized by others for misclassifying (Swindell et al., 1984; Wertz et al., 1984) or for forcing patients that may not fit a classical syndrome into a diagnostic category (Brookshire, 1997). Several materials that are required for administration are not included with the test and must be obtained separately.

WHAT IS THE TEST BEST SUITED FOR?

The WAB allows a reasonable sampling of an aphasic patient's language abilities on a variety of tasks in a fairly short time. Its classification system should be used cautiously.

Porch Index of Communicative Ability

General Description

SUBTESTS

The PICA consists of 18 subtests sampling *speaking, understanding spoken commands, reading, writing, object manipulation, visual matching,* and *copying abstract forms.* Each subtest consists of 10 items involving 10 objects that are used throughout the 18 subtests. The objects used are a toothbrush, cigarette, pen, knife, fork, quarter, pencil, matches, key, and comb. Internal consistency among subtests is enhanced by the use of these same objects across subtests and further by the use of the same scoring system for each subtest. In addition, because the same objects are used throughout the battery, responses based on recall of recent linguistic information are minimized by task ordering. Early in the examination, minimal linguistic information regarding the objects is provided by the examiner, with maximum information provided later in the test. A number of shortened versions of the PICA have been proposed and studied. For example, DiSimoni et al. (1975) questioned whether an abbreviated version would yield an overall score (grand mean of the 18 subtest means) comparable to the complete test. Using a stepwise regression analysis of 222 administrations of the complete PICA, they noted that only 10 subtests and five objects are needed to achieve the same overall score obtained from the complete test. Similar findings have been noted for two other short versions (DiSimoni et al., 1980). In another shortened version that used five objects (Phillips & Halpin, 1978), comparable reliability was noted, but this version was less sensitive to recovery beyond 4 weeks than the complete PICA (Lincoln & Ells, 1980).

INTENT
Porch developed the PICA to provide what he perceived to be lacking in other aphasia batteries at the time: a sensitive and reliable measurement of the degree of deficit and amount of recovery. Measurement of change is based on a multidimensional scoring system that is purported to be sensitive to subtle differences between aphasic behaviors.

TIME FOR ADMINISTRATION
Porch has reported that the PICA requires approximately 1 hour, on average, to administer, with a range of 22 to 143 minutes.

SCORING
In an effort to maximize the likelihood that the patient is assessed in the same way each time the test is presented, administration is restricted to fairly rigid guidelines prescribed in the manuals. These guidelines include exactly what the clinician is to say to the patient during the administration of each task; standard test conditions, such as a distraction-free testing environment, prescribed seating arrangement, specific arrangement of the testing objects, and specified procedures for each task; consistent order of task presentation; and completion of the battery in one testing session.

The multidimensional scoring system is probably the PICA's most unique feature. The system consists of a 16-point scale designed to quantify several dimensions of aphasic responses. The multidimensional nature of the scoring system is descriptive in that it reflects degrees of correctness and incorrectness, thus providing more quantitative information than plus-minus scores. The system is based on five dimensions of patient responses:

1. Accuracy (degree of correctness)
2. Responsiveness (ease with which an appropriate response is elicited)
3. Completeness of response (extent to which the task is carried out in its entirety)
4. Promptness (time required to respond)
5. Efficiency (motoric facility)

TABLE 4.2 Porch Index of Communicative Abilities scoring categories

Score	Category	Dimensional characteristics
16	Complex	Accurate, responsive, complex, prompt, efficient
15	Complete	Accurate, responsive, complete, prompt, efficient
14	Distorted	Accurate, responsive, complete or complex, prompt, distorted
13	Complete–delayed	Accurate, responsive, complete or complex, delayed
12	Incomplete	Accurate, responsive, incomplete, prompt
11	Incomplete–delayed	Accurate, responsive, incomplete, delayed
10	Corrected	Accurate, self-corrected
9	Repeated	Accurate, after instructions are repeated
8	Cued	Accurate after cue is given
7	Related	Inaccurate, almost accurate
6	Error	Inaccurate attempt at the task item
5	Intelligible	Comprehensible but not an attempt at the task item
4	Unintelligible	Incomprehensible but undifferentiated
3	Minimal	Incomprehensible and undifferentiated
2	Attention	No response, but patient attends to the tester
1	No response	No response, no awareness of task

These dimensions are combined into a rank order of response accuracy shown in Table 4.2, with 16 representing the most adequate response and 1 the least. Responses between 16 and 8 would represent correct responses in a plus-minus system, whereas 7 through 1 would be incorrect. Each of the patient's 180 responses (18 subtests of 10 items) is assigned one of these scores during administration of the PICA. In the 1981 revision of the test, Porch added diacritical markings to increase the precision of recording a patient's behavior.

MATERIALS NEEDED FOR ADMINISTRATION
To administer the PICA, the following are needed:

1. Porch Index of Communicative Ability (Porch, 1981a)
2. *Administration, Scoring, and Interpretation, Volume II*, 3rd edition (Porch, 1981b)
3. Ten test objects
4. Scoring and summary sheets

Normative Information (Standardization)
The PICA has been recognized for its norms and reliability, determined during development of the test. The test was developed over a 6-year period beginning in 1959.

POPULATIONS
Interpretation of test performance is facilitated by converting raw scores into percentiles that indicate degree of deficit with respect to a large sam-

ple of left-hemisphere–damaged aphasic subjects (280 in 1971, 357 in 1981). Porch's sampling of the aphasic population was purposefully designed to be reflective of those aphasic patients in the typical clinical caseload in terms of age, race, sex, education, occupation, and etiology. A percentile table is also included based on a sample of 100 bilaterally brain-damaged subjects (Porch, 1981b). Normative data for the PICA are also available for 130 normal subjects (Duffy et al., 1976) and 111 right-hemisphere–damaged patients (Deal et al., 1979) but are not available in the PICA manual.

INTERPRETATION OF SCORES

The numbers assigned to each response are averaged at different levels and the means recorded on the score sheet. The mean scores are used for determining degree of deficit, summarizing patterns of deficit, and making predictions of subsequent performance. The 10 responses for each task are averaged to provide a mean response level for each subtest. In the 1967 version, subtest means are averaged to provide mean response levels in the gestural, verbal, and graphic categories. The 1981 version permits interpretation with seven categories: verbal, pantomime, reading, auditory, visual, writing, and copying. The administration and interpretation manual provides tables for translating raw scores into percentile scores.

PROFILES

Mean scores reflect general degrees of deficit in various language functions, and the pattern of these deficits may be indicative of different disorders. Attempts have been made to determine whether profiles from the PICA might reflect different syndromes of aphasia. Porch (1971) described a profile for "aphasia with impaired verbal monitoring" that corresponds to Wernicke's aphasia. Porch (1978) has also proposed hypothetical relationships between functions isolated in specific subtests and different regions within the left hemisphere theoretically responsible for these functions. Six patterns were proposed and related to six regions of the brain. PICA profiles have also been used to distinguish among aphasia, apraxia, and dysarthria (Porch, 1971; Porch, 1978). Profiles from patients with diffuse bilateral brain damage have been described (Porch, 1971; Porch, 1978; Watson, 1978; Wertz, 1978), as well as cases of neurosis and psychosis, in which there is no brain damage, and cases of malingering, in which aphasia is feigned (Porch & Porec, 1977; Porec & Porch, 1977).

The PICA has been used extensively as an objective measure of recovery. It yields a single summarizing score that can be treated statistically to represent changes in single subtest-related functions, response categories, and overall language function. Mean scores are used as the basis for predicting later levels of function. The overall score (grand mean of 18 subtest means) is a single indicator of the amount of recovery made by an aphasic patient. The overall score is considered to be the most reliable of the mean scores because it reflects performance on all 180 items of the test. A variety of analyses have been suggested for predicting recovery. The "high-low gap" is one method of prediction and is based on the difference between the averages of the nine highest subtest scores and nine lowest subtest scores. This "gap" is what Porch referred to as the dynamic range of a patient's performance at any point during the period of recovery. The high percentile represents the patient's potential for overall recovery—that is, the patient's best performance soon after onset is considered to be an indication of potential for maximum overall recovery 5–6 months later.

The high overall prediction method is a second approach in which the overall score at 1 month postonset is converted into its corresponding high score in the table. That high score is used to derive the predicted overall score at 6 months postonset. This method is consistent with the theory that the initial high scores represent the upper limit of the dynamic range.

A third technique involves the peak-mean difference score, another measure of variance reflecting a dynamic range. The peak-mean difference is derived with a formula using the differences between the highest score and the mean score of each subtest. The use of such scores to predict recovery should be done with caution, and test scores may need to be supplemented with data related to other factors to maximize statistical predictions of recovery (Porch et al., 1980).

Theoretical Biases of Authors

According to Porch (1994), a brain injury results in a reduced capacity to store, switch, monitor, and perform many of the other steps necessary for the brain to receive, assimilate, and send information. Because these processes cannot be observed directly, they must be assessed by presenting the patient with a set of standard tasks, stimuli, and test conditions and carefully recording the response characteristics of the patient.

Validity, Reliability, and Sensitivity

Prescribed administration procedures and a carefully defined scoring system contribute to the PICA's demonstrated high reliability. Analysis of content validity of the PICA indicates that most of 18 subtests sample language function in the absence of communicative contexts, suggesting that the PICA is a test of language but not of communication per se (Davis, 1983). The PICA has been noted to have strong criterion-related validity with respect to other tests of aphasia (Holland, 1980; Keenan & Brassell, 1975; Sanders & Davis, 1978) but falls short of equivalent validity with respect to natural communicative function in daily life (Holland, 1980). Validity of the PICA's multidimensional scoring system has been investigated with respect to whether this scale truly represents a hierarchy of behavior—that is, whether it is truly an ordinal scale. Findings indicated that the scale indeed represents different levels of communicative accuracy and efficiency, but that the nature of the scale's ordinality may not correspond to other ways of ranking the acceptability of communicative behaviors (Duffy & Dale, 1977; McNeil et al., 1975). Duffy and Dale (1977) concluded that the PICA's scoring system functions as an interval scale and, therefore, the means can be used statistically with confidence.

Clinical Use
STRENGTHS
Strengths of the PICA include a thorough description of patient performances, reliability, indications for treatment planning, and opportunities for inter- and intrasubtest comparisons.

WEAKNESSES
Weaknesses of the PICA include limited sampling of communicative tasks, lack of measures to detect mild to subtle impairments in the auditory modality, the need for intensive training to insure validity, and reliability. (Porch has recommended at least 40 hours of training, including extensive scoring practice, before clinical use of the battery.)

WHAT IS THE TEST BEST SUITED FOR?
PICA is most appropriate for moderately aphasic patients who are medically stable and can meaningfully participate in an assessment session of 60–90 minutes in duration. It is excellent for quantifying language recovery.

Supplemental Tests for Aphasia

All of the aphasia batteries previously discussed are by design comprehensive in nature—that is, they test language in all four modalities. Consequently, some of these batteries—with the possible exception of the MTDDA—may not permit in-depth examination of all modalities. Therefore, a number of modality-specific supplemental tests have been developed. These tests examine a modality more thoroughly in an effort to delineate subtle problems in the mildly impaired individual or spared capabilities in the severely impaired individual. Such information has obvious relevance for treatment planning. Four supplemental tests of aphasia are described in this section:

1. Revised Token Test (RTT)
2. Boston Naming Test (BNT)
3. Test of Adolescent/Adult Word Finding (TAWF)
4. Reading Comprehension Battery for Aphasia (RCBA-2)

Revised Token Test
General Description
SUBTESTS
The RTT has 10 subtests of commands that differ in length and complexity. For example, subtest I consists of commands like, "Touch the black circle," whereas subtest X contains commands like, "Touch the big black square unless you have touched the little red circle."

INTENT
The RTT is designed to provide a sensitive, quantifiable assessment of auditory processing inefficiencies associated with brain damage, aphasia, and certain language and learning disabilities.

TIME FOR ADMINISTRATION
No information about the time needed for administration is included in the manual, but clinical experience suggests that the time needed can

TABLE 4.3   Revised token scoring

Correct

15	Complete	Response to individual unit within a command is prompt, without mediation tactics or extra information, and complete.
14	Vocal–subvocal rehearsal	Response is comparable to 15, except for the vocal or subvocal rehearsing of a portion of a command, but is done without unusual processing time.
13	Delay	Response produced as a complete response (15), but requires additional processing time to complete.
12	Immediacy	Response to which the individual is unable to mediate the command in any form and unable to use additional processing time to respond. Individual touches first token before the tester finishes giving the command.
11	Self-correction	Response is initially incorrect but is corrected without external feedback.
10	Reversal	Response in which any one set of units in a two-part command is reversed from the order in which they are verbally presented.
9	Repeat	Response after the repeated command statement.
8	Cue	Response after a repeat, for which the individual required more information because he or she did the wrong task, rejected the command, did not respond for 30 seconds, or requested a repeat.

Incorrect

7	Error	Response to an entire command or a unit within a command is incorrect and does not justify a repeat or cue.
6	Perseveration	Response to a command that is incorrect that is also identical to one preceding it.
5	Intelligible/rejection	Response that is intelligible or a rejection.
4	Unintelligible (differentiated)	Response that could not necessarily be judged to be an attempt at the task but is clearly different from other unintelligible responses.
3	Unintelligible (perseveration)	Response similar to 4 but is undifferentiated from previous unintelligible tasks.
2	Omission	Response in which one part of a two-part command was omitted.
1	No response	Individual does not respond.

Source: From M. R. McNeil, & T. E. Prescott, (1978). *Revised Token Test*. Baltimore: University Park Press.

range from 15 minutes to more than an hour, depending on the response latency of the individual being tested. To shorten administration and scoring time, Arvedson et al. (1985) investigated whether a shorter version could be used reliably and suggested that using the first five items in each subtest could reliably predict the overall score on the longer version.

SCORING

Each item is scored on each element of the command using a 15-point scoring system based on that of the PICA (Table 4.3). The number of elements ranges from three to eight, depending on the complexity of the command. The score for each item is the mean of its element scores. The score for each subtest is the mean of the element scores for the subtest.

The overall score is the mean of all subtest scores. Additionally, 11 linguistic element scores can be computed. Because of all the computations that are required, scoring can take 40–50 minutes.

MATERIALS NEEDED FOR ADMINISTRATION
To administer the RTT, the following are needed:

1. Administration manual
2. Scoring forms
3. Tokens

Normative Information (Standardization)

POPULATIONS
The standardization sample included 90 non–brain-damaged adults, 30 adults with left-hemisphere brain damage, and 30 adults with right-hemisphere brain damage, aged 20–80 years.

INTERPRETATION OF SCORES
Subtest scores and the overall score can be compared with percentile ranks of non–brain-damaged, left-hemisphere–damaged, and right-hemisphere–damaged individuals. The authors state that the RTT directly measures auditory short-term memory, comprehension of various sentence types, comprehension of specific vocabulary items, and comprehension of semantic relations. They suggest that examination of scores and profiles can provide insight into cognitive processes such as a set to attend, sustained and selective auditory attention, short-term memory, and temporal sequencing (McNeil & Prescott, 1978).

PROFILES
The authors provide theoretical performance profiles that they suggest are consistent with a number of cognitive processing impairments—namely, problems with increasing stimulus length, fatigue, short-term storage deficits, specific linguistic deficits, and intermittent auditory imperception (Hageman et al., 1982; McNeil & Hageman, 1979; McNeil & Prescott, 1978).

Theoretical Biases of Authors

The authors state that they designed the test to be clinically applicable in terms of differential diagnosis and ability to finitely describe patterns of auditory disorders. They propose theoretical performance profiles (described in the section Interpretation of Scores), which they suggest correspond to different patterns of auditory processing deficit (McNeil & Prescott, 1978).

Validity, Reliability, and Sensitivity

When constructing the test, the authors paid careful attention to such important psychometric dimensions as range of subtest difficulty, number of items per subtest, stimulus selection, and task selection. Moderate correlations were found between the RTT overall score and the PICA overall score for 23 aphasic subjects. Test-retest, intrascorer, and interscorer reliability results ranged from 0.90 to 0.99 for three examiners who had each received 24 hours of training on the multidimensional scoring system. Analysis of variance procedures showed that normal subjects scored significantly better than subjects with brain damage, and that the right-brain–damaged group scored significantly better than the left-brain–damaged group. The authors urged caution in using the test to differentiate right versus left brain damage, however, because these results are based on a small number of brain-damaged subjects (McNeil & Prescott, 1978).

Clinical Use

STRENGTHS

The RTT is able to detect mild auditory comprehension impairments that standardized aphasia batteries do not.

WEAKNESSES

The test requires a large expenditure of time to administer and to score, considering that it only provides information on one aspect of language ability. Although the authors propose theoretical profiles for different patterns of auditory processing impairments, there is little evidence that these profiles reflect actual patterns of impairment in brain-damaged people.

WHAT IS THE TEST BEST SUITED FOR?

The test is most appropriate for revealing mild auditory comprehension impairments. Because administering the first five items from each subtest was shown to reliably predict scores from the full version, using the shorter version of the test saves both administration and scoring time.

Boston Naming Test
General Description

SUBTESTS

The BNT is a picture-naming test consisting of 60 pictures (black and white line drawings), ordered from easiest to most difficult (i.e., "bed" to "abacus") with regard to word familiarity (frequency of occurrence).

INTENT

The BNT is one of several freestanding tests for assessing naming in brain-damaged adults described in the literature. Like the other tests of naming, the BNT is designed to sample naming abilities in greater depth than is typically accomplished in comprehensive aphasia batteries. For example, the visual confrontation naming subtest of the BDAE (Goodglass & Kaplan, 1983b) contains only six items in each of six categories, many of them easy, high-frequency words. The pictured items used in the BNT were selected to eliminate items that might have alternative acceptable names.

TIME FOR ADMINISTRATION

Depending on the patient's responsiveness and level of severity, time required to administer the BNT is typically fewer than 30 minutes.

SCORING

When the BNT is administered, each response is scored for latency, correctness, and whether a cue was given. A patient who appears not to recognize an object is provided with a function cue. If a response does not occur in 20 seconds, a phonemic cue is presented. It is recommended that a clinician begin with item 30 (i.e., harmonica) for adults but work backward if middle items are too difficult. Testing stops after six consecutive failures. The total score is derived from the total correct, with a maximum of 60.

To administer the BNT, the following materials are needed:

1. BNT manual (which includes administration instructions and pictures)
2. Response scoring booklet (which includes norms)

Normative Information (Standardization)
Norms are provided for a variety of normal children and adults, and aphasic adults (Kaplan et al., 1983).

POPULATIONS
Included in the response scoring booklet are norms for 30 non–brain-injured children (kindergarten to grade 5), 84 normal adults (aged 18–59 years), and 82 aphasic adults (at six levels of aphasic severity).

INTERPRETATION OF SCORES
The score summary at the end of the scoring booklet gives

1. Items correct without assistance
2. Number of stimulus cues given
3. Number correct after a stimulus cue
4. Number of phonemic cues given
5. Number correct after a phonemic cue

The total correct is the sum of items (1) and (2). The total score is the total correct plus credit for all items preceding the first item failed.

PROFILES
No profiles are described for the BNT.

Theoretical Biases of Authors
Two of the authors of the BNT, Kaplan and Goodglass, also authored the BDAE. Consequently, the theoretical biases reflected in the BDAE are comparable for the BNT.

Validity, Reliability, and Sensitivity
Scores from the BNT have been correlated with subtest scores and rating scales from the BDAE (Goodglass & Kaplan, 1983b). These include aphasia severity rating with visual confrontation naming and responsive naming, and with the finger naming subsection of the spatial-quantitative battery. According to Goodglass and Kaplan (1983b), the BNT does not correlate with the WAIS Verbal IQ nor with the vocabulary subtest of the WAIS. Moderate correlations (i.e., in the 0.60s) were observed with the oral word reading and oral sentence reading tasks. Other correlations with the BDAE subtests are relatively low.

Clinical Use
STRENGTHS
This test is quick and easy to administer. The BNT is also reportedly useful for detecting mild word-retrieval problems in individuals with dementia or children with developmental delays (Goodglass & Kaplan, 1983b).

WEAKNESSES

The BNT manual provides brief instructions for administering the BNT and scoring responses, but neither administration nor scoring instructions appear explicit enough to ensure interexaminer or test-retest reliability, and the manual does not report either (Brookshire, 1997). Nicholas and associates (1989) published more detailed procedures for administering and scoring the BNT, together with intrajudge and interjudge reliability results for those more detailed procedures.

WHAT IS THE TEST BEST SUITED FOR?

The BNT is most appropriate for mild to moderately aphasic patients.

Test of Adolescent/Adult Word Finding
General Description

SUBTESTS

Subtests of TAWF include picture naming—nouns, sentence completion naming, description naming, picture naming—verbs, category naming, and comprehension assessment.

INTENT

The intent of the TAWF is to assess word-finding skills in adolescents and adults using systematic test procedures and naming tasks.

TIME FOR ADMINISTRATION

The author estimates that the complete test should take 30 minutes to administer. There is a brief test that can be administered in approximately 15 minutes.

SCORING

All items are scored for accuracy. Responses to pictured nouns are also scored for speed. Correct responses receive a score of 1, whereas incorrect responses are recorded verbatim and receive a score of 0. Self-corrections are scored as incorrect, but visual misperceptions are not penalized. Appendices in the administration manual provide lists of acceptable and unacceptable substitutions for each item. Response time can be estimated or measured to the nearest hundredth of a second from a tape recording. If estimated response times are used, the examiner judges whether a response time is more or less than 4 seconds. The presence of gestures or extra verbalizations are recorded in the response booklet.

MATERIALS NEEDED FOR ADMINISTRATION

To administer the TAWF, the following materials are needed:

1. Test book
2. Response booklet
3. Administration, scoring, and interpretation manual

If the optional actual item response time measurement is used, an audio tape recorder, blank audio cassette, and a stopwatch with digital display that records time to hundredths of a second are also needed.

Normative Information (Standardization)

POPULATIONS

The norming sample consisted of 1,200 adolescents in grades 7–12 and 553 adults aged 20–80 years residing in 21 states (German, 1990a). Data from the 1980 U.S. Census were used to ensure adequate representation on a number of important demographic variables.

INTERPRETATION OF SCORES

A total raw score is obtained by adding scores of the five naming subtests. It is then converted to a standard score or a percentile rank. Standard errors of measurements for standard scores are provided, and confidence ranges can be calculated (German, 1990b).

PROFILES

By plotting the standard score against the response time average (for estimated or actual response times), a subject can be placed in one of four profiles:

1. Fast and inaccurate namer
2. Slow and inaccurate namer
3. Fast and accurate namer
4. Slow and accurate namer

The author states that these profiles are descriptive in nature and are not intended to imply underlying etiologies. Additionally, the examiner can analyze errors according to substitution type and note whether gestures or "extra verbalizations" accompanied or substituted for responses (German, 1990b).

Theoretical Biases of Authors

The author presents a brief review of research about word-finding problems in adult aphasia, learning disabilities, reading disorders, language disorders, and fluency disorders. This review is primarily concerned with studies that have documented the presence of word-finding problems in the context of those disorders and variables that may affect word retrieval (German, 1990b). The author does not discuss possible processes of word retrieval or theorize about the causes of word-finding problems.

Validity, Reliability, and Sensitivity

Preliminary field testing resulted in a final version that includes only items that at least 95% of the standardization sample comprehended. Internal consistency as measured by the Kuder-Richardson statistic was 0.85. Test-retest reliability for 30 normal adults yielded a correlation of 0.85 for accuracy and 0.72 for average item response time. Studies of concurrent validity for 30 normal seventh- and eighth-graders yielded moderate correlations between the TAWF and the BNT ($r = 0.66$) and for the TAWF and the Upper Extension of the Expressive One-Word Picture Vocabulary Test ($r = 0.62$). Eighteen aphasic adults scored significantly more poorly than 18 normal adults on the complete and brief versions of the TAWF (German, 1990a).

Clinical Use

STRENGTHS

The TAWF measures a number of naming abilities—specifically, naming verbs, description naming, and category naming—that are not typically investigated in other standardized tests. The TAWF also assesses the subject's comprehension of each missed item, thus allowing the examiner to assess whether an error truly represents a word-retrieval problem, or whether the item was not in the subject's vocabulary. The large sample of normal adults aged 20–80 years on whom the norms are based is also a strength of this test.

WEAKNESSES

The TAWF does not allow credit for self-corrections and thus seems to penalize many aphasic individuals. However, examiners can easily compensate for this by noting self-corrections on the test form and discussing the number of items that were self-corrected when reporting the test results.

WHAT IS THE TEST BEST SUITED FOR?

This test provides a relatively quick standardized method to assess a range of naming abilities. Because it provides norms to 80 years, it is presumably a more reliable test to use with adults aged 59–80 years than is the BNT, which does not provide norms for individuals in that age group.

Reading Comprehension Battery for Aphasia
General Description

SUBTESTS

The second edition of the Reading Comprehension Battery for Aphasia (RCBA-2) (LaPointe & Horner, 1988) is composed of 10 core subtests, each containing 10 items. Each subtest is scored for accuracy and completion time, which are reported in raw scores. Subtests I, II, and III all involve single-word comprehension with *visual confusions, auditory confusions,* and *semantic confusions,* respectively. Subtest IV involves having the patient read short phrases or passages and answer questions of a *functional* nature. In subtest V, *synonyms,* the patient must select a synonym for the stimulus word from a group of three words. In subtests VI and VII, *sentence comprehension* and *paragraph comprehension,* the patient reads a sentence or paragraph and points to one of three pictures that best depicts the sentence or paragraph. Subtests VIII and IX, *paragraphs—factual* and *inferential comprehension,* are presented together. The patient is required to read a paragraph and answer two questions involving factual comprehension and two questions involving inferential comprehension of the passage. Subtest X, *morpho-syntactic reading,* requires the patient to read three sentences that increase in syntactic complexity and to select a sentence that goes with the picture.

The RCBA-2 also contains seven supplemental subtests that were not available in the original version of the battery. The seven supplemental subtests contain between five and 40 test items. Subtest XI, *letter discrimination,* requires the patient to state whether various combinations of letter pairs are the same or different. Subtests XII and XIII, *letter naming* and *letter recognition*, consist of full visual field, right visual field, and left visual field arrangements of letters with "X" in the center field for orientation. In subtest XII, the patient is required to point to and name the letters. In subtest XIII, the patient is required to point to the letters on the page that match the examiner's spoken word. Subtest XIV, *lexical decision*, presents the patient with three consonant-vowel-consonant trigrams: Two are nonsense words and one is a real English word that the patient is to identify. In subtest XV, *semantic categorization*, a category name and a word are presented, and the patient must indicate whether the words are associated. In subtests XVI and XVII, *oral reading — words* and *oral reading — sentences*, the patient is required to either read words of increasing length aloud, or read subject-verb-object sentences aloud.

INTENT
According to the authors, the RCBA-2 was designed to provide systematic evaluation of the nature and degree of reading impairment in adolescents and adults with aphasia. The original version of the RCBA was developed to meet a long-standing clinical need for a practical measure of reading comprehension with the nuances of aphasia in mind (LaPointe & Horner, 1988).

TIME FOR ADMINISTRATION
The core subtests of the RCBA-2 can be administered in approximately 1 hour.

SCORING
The examiner records each response in the appropriate section in the profile/summary record form. A correct response is given a 1; an incorrect response a 0. At the end of each subtest, the examiner records the amount of time the patient required to complete the subtest. In addition, all of the core subtests and many of the supplemental subtests require the examiner to write any incorrect responses in the space provided.

MATERIALS NEEDED FOR ADMINISTRATION
Administration of the RCBA-2 requires

1.   Picture books
2.   Profile/summary record form
3.   Wristwatch with a second hand

NORMATIVE INFORMATION (STANDARDIZATION)
The RCBA-2 manual contains no normative information.

POPULATIONS
The authors note that the RCBA-2 is a criterion-referenced rather than a norm-referenced measure. Consequently, the test manual contains no normative information.

INTERPRETATION OF SCORES
The RCBA-2 yields two types of scores: accuracy and speed scores. In addition, scores can be examined by clinicians in terms of quantity and quality. *Quantity* refers to the number of items the patient answers correctly as well as the time it takes for the patient to complete the test. *Quality* refers to the type of errors a patient makes. The range of com-

prehension tasks sampled and the linguistic controls guiding stimulus selections within the core subtests allow the examiner to ascertain level of performance overall, among subtests, and within subtests. Changes over time can be observed by differences in level of accuracy and by increases or decreases in the amount of time necessary to complete the test. This allows performance to be tracked on successive testings for the same individual. Changes in the degree of reading impairment that result from treatment or simply the passage of time can be quantified and documented (LaPointe & Horner, 1988).

Analysis of the quality of error (i.e., the pattern of predominant type) of silent reading comprehension deficit has clinical and theoretical implications. Several of the controls used in the selection of stimulus materials for the RCBA-2 emanate from literature on oral and silent reading deficits as well as from normative studies that are reviewed in the first chapter of the RCBA-2 manual. Included here are auditory, visual, and semantic factors; parts of speech; picturability; age of acquisition of picturable nouns; frequency of occurrence, imageability, and concreteness; length of word, phrase, or text; and morpho-syntax. The authors observe that clinicians interested in practical, effective, and theoretically sound intervention strategies must not only ask how much, and where, but also why performance breaks down. The clinician must then attempt to discover those mechanisms that relate to the particular type of impairment.

PROFILES

Space is provided on the profile/summary record form for (1) specifying pertinent information about the patient, (2) recording RCBA-2 subtest results in terms of raw score and total time, and (3) profiling the patient's RCBA-2 subtest performance. The examiner can graph the results of the 10 core subtests to provide an overview of strengths and weaknesses. In addition, a comment section is provided for the examiner to record patient-specific information, such as general attention and cooperation, head posture, visual scanning, and special testing requirements.

Theoretical Biases of Authors

Development of the RCBA and RCBA-2 was motivated by what the authors perceived as an unmet clinical need. Many of their aphasic clients had difficulties with reading, yet the nature of these reading problems had to be derived from performance on subtests of traditional aphasia batteries or from reading tests designed for use with children or adolescents. Many of the reading subtests of aphasia batteries seemed to be abbreviated and incomplete and did not address many of the characteristic problems of reading seen in aphasia. Further, the more general reading test batteries either contained material only marginally appropriate to adult reading interests or failed to account for some of the peculiarities of reading induced by nervous system damage. Construction of the RCBA-2 was guided by a body of literature on aphasia and on the reading process, and in particular by a small number of studies on reading problems in aphasia. Material was selected to be suitable to adult interests so that the test would not be demeaning. Items were also selected to satisfy the requirement of being at the least difficult vocabulary and reading levels. In the presence of reading difficulty at the word or sentence level, it is important to delineate the underlying reasons for the errors. The supplemental tasks are designed to evaluate prerequisite reading abilities and to identify intact modalities or spared strategies that might serve as the basis for hierarchic reading programs (Horner, 1980; Horner & Massey, 1986; Horner et al., 1989).

Validity, Reliability, and Sensitivity
Although no normative information or documentation of the RCBA-2's reliability and validity is included in the manual, some psychometric information on the core subtests is available elsewhere. No studies have been conducted with the RCBA supplemental subtests. Reliability and validity of the RCBA were investigated using two groups of aphasic patients (Van DeMark et al., 1982). Test-retest reliability was noted to be high; internal consistency reliability was similarly high, indicating a high degree of homogeneity within items and across individuals. Criterion-referenced validity of the RCBA was also investigated in the same study using two measures: the Gates Silent Reading Test and subtests from the PICA. The correlation coefficients were $r = 0.80$ for the Gates–RCBA scores and $r = 0.87$ for the PICA subtests–RCBA scores. These authors concluded that the RCBA has high levels of test stability, internal consistency, and validity. As an instrument for measuring reading comprehension in aphasia, the RCBA appears to be psychometrically sound (Van DeMark et al., 1982).

A second study of the RCBA (Pasternack & LaPointe, 1982) established the test-retest and intertester reliability and compared performance of aphasic subjects with nonaphasic adults and normal sixth-graders. For the 10 aphasic subjects, the test-retest reliability coefficient was 0.99. Intertester reliability was determined by comparing the scores of five subjects by four judges on 10 subtests. Results revealed agreement on 180 out of 200 judgments (90% agreement). Results for the nonaphasic subjects showed a high degree of ease in completing the battery.

Clinical Use
STRENGTHS
The RCBA-2 was the first commercially available test designed specifically to address acquired reading problems in aphasia. It is one of the most widely used supplemental tests of aphasia and assesses reading at a variety of levels, including functional reading (i.e., reading tasks encountered in daily living).

WEAKNESSES
Limited normative data are available. The RCBA has been criticized because of text independence in subtests VIII and IX (Nicholas et al., 1986). The problem—common to a number of aphasia test batteries—is that some items in the subtests involving paragraphs could be answered correctly beyond chance levels by aphasic and non–brain-damaged subjects who had not read the paragraphs to which test items referred. These subtests should be interpreted cautiously.

The RCBA-2 is most appropriate for a wide range of aphasic patients, mildly to severely impaired. It provides a good starting point for developing a therapy program for reading problems in aphasia.

Aphasia Tests for Special Purposes

In addition to these comprehensive aphasia batteries and supplemental tests for aphasia, there are also a number of testing instruments that were developed for specific populations or specific purposes. Two such tests are discussed in this section: the Boston Assessment of Severe Aphasia (BASA) and the CADL.

Boston Assessment of Severe Aphasia
General Description
SUBTESTS
The BASA is composed of 14 subtests or sections:

1. Social greetings and simple conversation
2. Personally relevant yes/no question pairs
3. Orientation to time and place
4. Bucco-facial praxis
5. Sustained "ah" and singing
6. Repetition, limb praxis
7. Comprehension of number symbols
8. Object naming
9. Action picture items
10. Comprehension of coin names
11. Famous faces
12. Emotional words, phrases, and symbols
13. Visuo-spatial items
14. Signature

INTENT
As stated by the authors, the BASA is a screening tool designed for the specific purpose of identifying and quantifying preserved abilities that might form the basis of a starting point for therapy for severely aphasic patients. The stimulus materials and tasks were selected on the basis of clinical and experimental evidence suggesting that these patients may retain the ability to process certain types of linguistic and paralinguistic information seldom probed in other aphasia measures (Helm-Estabrooks et al., 1989).

TIME FOR ADMINISTRATION
Most patients can complete this test in 30–40 minutes.

SCORING
Throughout the BASA, the patient's responses are scored for response modality (i.e., verbal, gestural, or both), communicative quality (i.e., rated on a 4-point scale, from refusal or rejection of the task to fully communi-

cative or correct response), perseveration (i.e., if the patient responds by repeating or continuing a response produced within the last five items or produces verbal stereotypies), and presence of affect (i.e., a verbal or gestural response produced with emotional affect). Patient performance is summarized in two types of scores: (1) scores pertaining to specific clusters of related BASA items, and (2) a total score computed by summing scores of all the items. The BASA consists of seven clusters of test items: auditory comprehension, praxis, oral-gestural expression, reading comprehension, gesture recognition, writing, and visuo-spatial tasks. The raw score for the item cluster is the number of items in that cluster for which the patient provided a fully communicative response in the modality specified. The BASA record form provides a section to sum and record scores on BASA item clusters. The BASA total score is the sum of the item cluster raw scores. Each cluster contributes equally to the BASA total score; no attempt has been made to weight the contribution of individual items or item clusters to the BASA total score.

MATERIALS NEEDED FOR ADMINISTRATION

All materials required for administration of the BASA are included in the test kit with the exception of four coins (quarter, dime, nickel, and penny). The BASA manual contains administration and scoring instructions as well as normative data.

Normative Information (Standardization)

The norms are based on a sample of more than 100 aphasic patients. These data are summarized in tables and included in the BASA manual.

POPULATIONS

The two groups of aphasic patients include 111 with severe aphasia and 47 diagnosed as globally aphasic.

INTERPRETATION OF SCORES

An intended goal of the BASA is to help determine whether a severe case of aphasia may be classified as *global*; thus, the separate table of norms is provided for the group of globally aphasic patients. This allows the clinician to compare the patient's obtained BASA score with the scores of either patients with severe aphasia or global aphasia.

PROFILES

No profiles are reported, but scores may be summarized by item clusters. BASA performance can be analyzed to identify the patient's response modality hierarchy by noting the percentage of responses in each modality that have at least partial communicative value. The information obtained from these analyses may then be used to design an individual treatment program that encourages further development of the patient's strongest response modality, using stimuli that elicit the most communicative responses (Pasternack & LaPointe, 1982).

Theoretical Biases of Authors

Based on their own clinical experience and the aphasia literature, the authors identified a number of factors observed to enhance the language performance of severely aphasic patients—emotionality, humor, music, gesture recognition and expression, drawing, and writing—and incorporated them into the BASA tasks. They also have attempted to control for the imprecision caused by such extrinsic factors as severe apraxia, perseveration, and hemiattentional deficits in visual perception. Finally, the authors note the importance of considering nonverbal responses (i.e., facial expression, vocal inflection, and gestures) in overall communicative functioning. Thus, any relevant aspect of the patient's behavior can provide quantifiable information for making a diagnosis on the basis of BASA performance.

Validity, Reliability, and Sensitivity
The psychometric aspects of the BASA have been carefully considered. With regard to content validity, moderate correlations were reported between the BASA item clusters and certain subtests of the BDAE, including the Aphasia Severity Rating Scale. The average interrater reliability was noted to be more than 90% for both the verbal and gestural scores.

Clinical Use
STRENGTHS
The BASA is easily administered in a short period of time. It is one of the only assessment batteries specifically designed for severe aphasia and has been carefully developed psychometrically.

WEAKNESSES
This test is not widely used at the current time. It is somewhat awkward to administer at bedside because of the variety of stimulus materials (i.e., objects and cards) needed to administer the test.

WHAT IS THE TEST BEST SUITED FOR?
The BASA is most appropriate for aphasic individuals with severe impairments in both comprehension and production of language.

Communicative Abilities in Daily Living
General Description
SUBTESTS
The CADL assesses communication activities in seven areas:

1. Reading, writing, and using numbers
2. Social interactions
3. Divergent communication
4. Contextual communication
5. Nonverbal communication
6. Sequential relationships
7. Humor/metaphor/absurdity

INTENT
The purpose of the test is to assess the functional communication skills of adults with neurogenic communication disorders and to provide information of a different nature than standardized aphasia batteries, which are typically designed to measure linguistic impairment rather than to assess residual functional communication abilities.

TIME FOR ADMINISTRATION

According to the authors, the test can be administered in approximately 30 minutes.

SCORING

Responses are scored as wrong (0), adequate (1), or correct (2). Any response that clearly conveys the appropriate message to the examiner, regardless of its linguistic accuracy or the modality used, is considered correct. Adequate responses are those that contain elements of the appropriate message but do not convey the message clearly or completely, or correct responses to items that the examiner had to repeat after 5 seconds because the patient did not respond initially. Wrong responses include frank errors, silence, jargon, stereotypies, and so forth. The manual contains examples of responses that would be scored at each level for each item.

MATERIALS NEEDED FOR ADMINISTRATION

The following are needed for administration of the CADL:

1. Examiner manual
2. Picture book
3. Examiner record book
4. Patient response form

Additional requirements are a pencil, access to a working telephone, phone numbers typed onto a directory label, four $1 bills, and four quarters.

Normative Information (Standardization)

POPULATIONS

The second edition was normed on 175 English-speaking adults between the ages of 20 and 96 with neurogenic communication disorders, primarily from stroke or traumatic brain injury. They were drawn from 17 states. Demographic data derived from the sample were compared with data from the U.S. Bureau of the Census published in 1997, revealing that the sample was nationally representative.

INTERPRETATION OF SCORES

Raw scores can be converted into stanine scores and percentile scores based on performance of the norming sample of neurogenically disordered individuals.

PROFILES

Profiles for performance of global, mixed, Wernicke's, Broca's, and anomic aphasic subjects were provided in the manual for the first edition of the test, but have been eliminated from the second edition.

Theoretical Biases of Authors

The authors point out that most standardized aphasia batteries use language tasks that are not representative of normal communicative interactions, and that the testing procedures themselves seek to minimize the contextual cues that are present in every communicative situation. Accordingly, although performance on such tests may provide important information about the nature and severity of linguistic impairment, it does not provide information about how well or poorly individuals use their residual abilities in everyday interactions to communicate. If improving individuals' communicative ability is the ultimate goal of therapy, the authors argue that it is important to have reliable information about communicative, as well as linguistic, ability.

VALIDITY, RELIABILITY, AND SENSITIVITY

Criterion-related validity was established by a moderate correlation ($r = 0.66$, $p < .01$) between performance on the CADL-2 and performance on the WAB. Content validity was established through item-discrimination analysis. Internal consistency was demonstrated via Cronbach's alpha procedure, which yielded a coefficient alpha of 0.93. Test-retest reliability coefficients were high for the raw score and the stanine scores. Interexaminer reliability was 0.99. The mean stanine and raw scores from groups of neurologically impaired and neurologically normal people were statistically different (Holland et al., 1999).

Clinical Use

STRENGTHS

This test is the only standardized instrument available that assesses an aphasic individual's ability to communicate in situations that resemble actual, common activities of daily living. It is extremely useful for obtaining an impression of how the individual is actually communicating outside the sometimes sterile clinical environment.

WEAKNESSES

The authors caution that the CADL-2 only addresses fundamental aspects of limitations that a communication disorder like aphasia might impose; it doesn't measure the extent of the restrictions on participating in a full social life. They also warn that it should be used cautiously in settings in which there are a large percentage of individuals with dementia.

WHAT IS THE TEST BEST SUITED FOR?

This test is most appropriate for determining how an individual probably communicates in "real life." It can identify communicative strengths and weaknesses, thus making important contributions to treatment planning.

Screening Tests for Aphasia

Practicing clinicians in acute medical settings are faced with increasingly shorter periods of time to conduct evaluations of individuals suspected to have aphasia. It is not uncommon for patients to be discharged to a nursing home, rehabilitation facility, or even home within 1 week postonset. Given such time constraints, administration of a complete test battery may not always be feasible. Many clinicians have opted to use screening tests designed for the purpose of a speedy assessment. Some of these tests are briefly described.

Sklar Aphasia Scale

The Sklar Aphasia Scale (Sklar, 1973) can be administered in approximately 1 hour. Each modality (i.e., speaking, understanding what is said, reading, and writing) is tested, with five subtests containing five items. A 5-point scoring system (0–4) is used, with 0 designating a normal response and 4 points an incorrect response. Higher scores indicate greater degrees of impairment.

Aphasia Language Performance Scales

The Aphasia Language Performance Scales (Keenan & Brassell, 1975) provide an informal standardized assessment in fewer than 30 minutes. Objects from the patient's room can be used for assessing comprehension and expression. Each modality is tested with four scales, each containing items of increasing difficulty.

Bedside Evaluation Screening Test

The Bedside Evaluation Screening Test (Fitch-West & Sands, 1987) comes in a portable kit composed of a magnetic display board, objects, and summary report forms. Test administration requires approximately 20 minutes, including completion of the report form. Subtests include *auditory comprehension, reading, naming, repetition,* and *conversation*.

Acute Aphasia Screening Protocol

The Acute Aphasia Screening Protocol (Crary et al., 1989) can be administered in 10 minutes and uses common objects consistently present in a patient's room, such as a TV, pillow, or window. The test begins with a brief look at attention and orientation followed by screening of auditory comprehension and basic expressive skills, including a rating of conversational style. Validity and reliability have been reported.

Conclusion

Treatment planning for aphasia is a highly complex process. The treatment planning process begins with an evaluation of the aphasic individual's communication strengths and weaknesses, using standardized and informal measures. Because each patient brings a diverse combination of factors to the clinical setting—apart from a communicative diagnosis and etiology—these must also be considered during the planning process. Such factors include age, motivation, vocational/educational history, and family support. Consideration of assessment findings without placing that information within the context of the individual's personal circumstances yields an intervention approach that is generic, impersonal, and ineffective. Further, such an approach to treatment planning most likely focuses on the impairment and disability levels as opposed to the handicap level.

For example, two individuals with similarly mild aphasia present with comparable communicative disabilities. Suppose that one individual is a greenskeeper and the other a school teacher. From that perspective, the relatively mild disability might be a minor handicap for the greenskeeper and a potentially devastating handicap for the teacher. The treatment approach for these two individuals should be very different, despite the fact that they both have mild aphasia.

The assessment tools selected to evaluate an individual with aphasia should not simply reflect the theoretical bias of the clinician. To a large extent, assessment tools should be determined by the idiosyncratic circumstances of each patient, not simply his or her communicative diagnosis.

References

Arvedson, J. C., McNeil, M. R., & West, T. L. (1985). Prediction of Revised Token Test: Overall, subtest, and linguistic unit scores by two shortened versions. *Clinics in Aphasiology, 15,* 57–63.

Borod, J. C., Goodglass, H., & Kaplan, E. (1980). Normative data on the Boston Diagnostic Aphasia Examination, Parietal Lobe Battery, and the Boston Naming Test. *Journal of Clinical Neuropsychology, 2,* 209–215.

Brookshire, R. H. (1997). *Introduction to neurogenic communication disorders* (5th ed.). St. Louis, MO: Mosby.

Crary M. A., Haak, N. J., & Malinsky, A. E. (1989). Preliminary psychometric evaluation of an acute aphasia screening protocol. *Aphasiology, 3,* 611–618.

Davis, G. A. (1983). *A survey of adult aphasia.* Englewood Cliffs, NJ: Prentice-Hall, Inc.

Deal, J. L., Deal, L., Wertz, R. T., Kitselman, K., & Dwyer, C. (1979). Right hemisphere PICA percentiles: Some speculations about aphasia. In R. H. Brookshire (Ed.), *Clinical aphasiology conference proceedings* (pp. 30–37). Minneapolis: BRK Publishers.

DiSimoni, F. G., Keith, R. L., & Darley, F. L. (1980). Prediction of PICA overall score by short versions of the test. *Journal of Speech and Hearing Research, 23,* 511–516.

DiSimoni, F. G., Keith, R. L., Holt, D. L., & Darley, F. L. (1975). Practicality of shortening the Porch Index of Communicative Ability. *Journal of Speech and Hearing Research, 18,* 491–497.

Duffy, J. R., & Dale, B. J. (1977). The PICA scoring scale: Do its statistical shortcomings cause clinical problems? In R. H. Brookshire (Ed.), *Clinical aphasiology conference proceedings* (pp. 290–296). Minneapolis: BRK Publishers.

Duffy, J. R., Keith, R. L., Shane, H., & Podraza, B. L. (1976). Performance of normal (non-brain-injured) adults on the Porch Index of Communicative Ability. In R. H. Brookshire (Ed.), *Clinical aphasiology conference proceedings* (pp. 32–42). Minneapolis: BRK Publishers.

Fitch-West, J., & Sands, E. S. (1987). *Bedside Evaluation Screening Test.* Rockville, MD: Aspen.

Frattali, C., Thompson, C. K., Holland, A., Wohl, C.B., & Ferketic, M.M. (1995). *Functional assessment of communication skills for adults (ASHA FACS).* Rockville, MD: American Speech-Language Hearing Association.

German, D. J. (1990a). *Test of Adolescent/Adult Word Finding: Administration, scoring and interpretation manual.* Austin, TX: Pro-Ed.

German, D. J. (1990b). *Test of Adolescent/Adult Word Finding: Technical manual.* Austin, TX: Pro-Ed.

Giles, G. M. (1994). Functional assessment and intervention. In M. A. J. Finlayson & S. H. Garner (Eds.), *Brain injury rehabilitation: Clinical considerations.* Baltimore: Williams & Wilkins, 124–156.

Goodglass, H., & Kaplan, E. (1972). *The Boston Diagnostic Aphasia Examination.* Philadelphia: Lea & Febiger.

Goodglass, H., & Kaplan, E. (1983a). *The assessment of aphasia and related disorders* (2nd ed.). Philadelphia: Lea & Febiger.

Goodglass, H., & Kaplan, E. (1983b). *The Boston Diagnostic Aphasia Examination*. Philadelphia: Lea & Febiger.

Goodglass, H., Quadfasel, F. A., & Timberlake, W. H. (1964). Phrase length and the type and severity of aphasia. *Cortex, 1,* 133–153.

Hageman, C. F., McNeil, M. R., Rucci-Zimmer, S., & Cariski, D. (1982). The reliability of patterns of auditory processing deficits: Evidence from the Revised Token Test. In R. H. Brookshire (Ed.), *Clinical aphasiology conference proceedings* (pp. 230–234). Minneapolis: BRK Publishers.

Harvey, R., & Jellinek, H. (1979). *Patient Evaluation Conference System (PECS)*. Wheaton, IL: Marianjoy Rehabilitation Center.

Heinemann, A. (1993). *Rehabilitation Institute of Chicago Functional Assessment Scales (RIC-FAS)*. Chicago: Rehabilitation Institute of Chicago.

Helm-Estabrooks, N., Ramsberger, G., Morgan, A. R., & Nicholas, M. (1989). *Boston Assessment of Severe Aphasia: Manual*. Chicago: Applied Symbolix.

Holland, A. L. (1980). *Communicative abilities in daily living*. Baltimore: University Park Press.

Holland, A., Frattali, C., & Fromm, D. (1999). *Communicative Abilities in Daily Living* (2nd ed.). Austin, TX: Pro-Ed.

Horner, J. (1980). Visual agnostic misnaming: Treatment of a right CVA patient one year post onset. *Clinical Aphasiology, 10,* 316–330.

Horner, J., & Massey, E. W. (1986). Dynamic spelling alexia. *Journal of Neurology, Neurosurgery, and Psychiatry, 3,* 7–13.

Horner, J., Massey, E. W., Woodruff, W. W., Chase, K. N., & Dawson, D. W. (1989). Task dependent neglect: Computed tomography size and locus correlations. *Journal of Neurology Rehabilitation, 3,* 7–17.

Kaplan, E., Goodglass, H., & Weintraub, S. (1983). *The Boston Naming Test*. Philadelphia: Lea & Febiger.

Keenan, J. S., & Brassell, E. G. (1975). *Aphasia Language Performance Scales*. Murfreesboro, TN: Pinnacle Press.

Kertesz, A. (1979). *Aphasia and associated disorders: Taxonomy, localization, and recovery*. New York: Grune & Stratton.

Kertesz, A. (1982). *The Western Aphasia Battery*. New York: Grune & Stratton.

LaPointe, L. L., & Horner, J. (1988). *Reading Comprehension Battery for Aphasia, (2nd ed.) examiner's manual*. Austin, TX: Pro-Ed.

Lincoln, N. B., & Ells, P. (1980). A shortened version of the PICA. *British Journal of Disorders of Communication, 15,* 183–187.

Linebaugh, C. W. (1979). Assessing the assessments: The adequacy of standardized tests of aphasia. *Clinics in Aphasiology, 9,* 8–22.

Lomas, J., Pickard, L., Bester, S., Elbard, S., Finlayson, A. & Zoghaib, C. (1989). The Communicative Effectiveness Index: Development and psychometric evaluation of a functional communication measure for adult aphasia. *Journal of Speech and Hearing Disorders, 54,* 113–124.

McNeil, M. R., & Hageman, C. F. (1979). Auditory processing deficits in aphasia evidenced on the Revised Token Test: Incidence and prediction of across subtest and across item within subtest patterns. In R. H. Brookshire (Ed.), *Clinical aphasiology conference proceedings* (pp. 47–69). Minneapolis: BRK Publishers.

McNeil, M. R., & Prescott, T. E. (1978). *Revised Token Test*. Baltimore: University Park Press.

McNeil, M. R., Prescott, T. E., & Chang, E. C. (1975). A measure of PICA ordinality. In R. H. Brookshire (Ed.), *Clinical aphasiology conference proceedings* (pp. 113–124). Minneapolis: BRK Publishers.

Naeser, M. A., & Hayward, R. W. (1978). Lesion localization in aphasia with cranial computed tomography and the Boston Diagnostic Aphasia Exam. *Brain and Language, 2,* 363–368.

Nicholas, L. E., Brookshire, R. H., MacLennan, D. L., Schumacher, J. G., & Porrazzo, S. A. (1989). Revised administration and scoring procedures for the Boston Naming Test and norms for non-brain-damaged adults. *Aphasiology, 3,* 569–580.

Nicholas, L. E., MacLennan, D. L., & Brookshire, R. (1986). Validity of multiple-sentence reading comprehension tests for aphasic adults. *Journal of Speech and Hearing Disorders, 51,* 82–87.

Pasternack, K. F., & LaPointe, L. L. (1982). Aphasic-nonaphasic performance on the Reading Comprehension Battery for Aphasia (RCBA): Presentation at the annual convention of the American Speech-Language Hearing Association, Toronto, Canada.

Phillips, P. P., & Halpin, G. (1978). Language impairment evaluation in aphasic patients. *Archives of Physical Medicine and Rehabilitation, 59,* 327–329.

Porch, B. E. (1971). *Administration, scoring, and interpretation, Vol. II* (revised ed.). Palo Alto: Consulting Psychologists Press.

Porch, B. E. (1978). Profiles of aphasia: Test interpretation regarding localization of lesions. In R. H. Brookshire (Ed.), *Clinical aphasiology conference proceedings* (pp. 78–92). Minneapolis: BRK Publishers.

Porch, B. E. (1981a). *Porch Index of Communicative Ability*. Palo Alto: Consulting Psychologists Press.

Porch, B. E. (1981b). *Administration, scoring, and interpretation, Vol. II* (3rd ed.). Palo Alto: Consulting Psychologists Press.

Porch, B. E. (1994). Treatment of aphasia subsequent to the Porch Index of Communicative Ability (PICA). In R. Chapey (Ed.), *Language intervention strategies in adult aphasia* (3rd ed.) (pp. 178–183). Baltimore: Williams & Wilkins.

Porch, B. E, Collins, M., Wertz, R. T., & Friden, T. P. (1980). Statistical prediction of change in aphasia. *Journal of Speech and Hearing Research, 23,* 312–321.

Porch, B. E., & Porec, J. P. (1977). Medical-legal application of PICA results. In R. H. Brookshire (Ed.), *Clinical aphasiology conference proceedings* (pp. 302–309). Minneapolis: BRK Publishers.

Porec, J. P., & Porch, B. E. (1977). The behavioral characteristics of "simulated" aphasia. In R. H. Brookshire (Ed.), *Clinical aphasiology conference proceedings* (pp. 297–301). Minneapolis: BRK Publishers.

Powell, B. E., Bailey, S., & Clarke, E. (1980). A very short form of the Minnesota Aphasia Test. *British Journal of Social and Clinical Psychology, 19,* 189–194.

Powell, B. E., Clarke, E., & Bailey, S. (1979). Categories of aphasia: A cluster-analysis of Schuell test profiles. *British Journal of Disorders of Communication, 14,* 111–122.

Rancho Los Amigos Medical Center. (1993). *Rancho Rehabilitation Outcome Evaluation (RROE)*. Downey, CA: Author.

Sanders, S. B., & Davis, G. A. (1978). A comparison of the Porch Index of Communicative Ability and the Western Aphasia Battery. In R. H. Brookshire (Ed.), *Clinical aphasiology conference proceedings* (pp. 117–126). Minneapolis: BRK Publishers.

Sarno, M. T. (1969). *The Functional Communication Profile: Manual of directions (Rehabilitation monograph 42)*. New York: New York University Medical Center, Institute of Rehabilitation Medicine.

Schuell, H. M. (1965, 1972). *The Minnesota Test for Differential Diagnosis of Aphasia*. Minneapolis: University of Minnesota Press.

Schuell, H. M., Jenkins, J. J., & Carroll, J. B. (1962). A factor analysis of the Minnesota Test for the Differential Diagnosis of Aphasia. *Journal of Speech and Hearing Research, 5,* 349–369.

Schuell, H. M., Jenkins, J. J., & Jimenez-Pabon, E. (1965). *Aphasia in adults*. New York: Harper and Row.

Shewan, C. M., & Kertesz, A. Reliability and validity characteristics of the Western Aphasia Battery (WAB). *Journal of Speech, Language, and Hearing Research 45,* 308–324

Sklar, M. (1973). *Sklar Aphasia Scale* (revised ed.). Los Angeles: Western Psychological Services.

Starch, S., & Falltrick, E. (1990). The importance of home evaluation for brain injured clients: A team approach. *Cognitive Rehabilitation, 8,* 28–32.

State University of New York at Buffalo. (1990). *Functional Independence Measure (FIM) (Uniform data system for medical rehabilitation)*. Buffalo: Author.

Swindell, C. S., Holland, A. L., & Fromm, D. (1984). Classification of aphasia: WAB type versus clinical impression. In R. H. Brookshire (Ed.), *Clinical aphasiology conference proceedings* (pp. 48–54). Minneapolis: BRK Publishers.

Thompson, J., & Enderby, P. (1979). Is all your Schuell really necessary? *British Journal of Disorders of Communication, 14,* 195–201.

Van DeMark, A. A., Lemmer, C. J., & Drake, M. L. (1982). Measurement of reading comprehension in aphasia with the RCBA. *Journal of Speech and Hearing Disorders, 47,* 288–291.

Wallace, G. L. (1996). Management of aphasic individuals from culturally and linguistically diverse populations. In G. L. Wallace (Ed.), *Adult aphasia rehabilitation*. Boston: Butterworth–Heinemann.

Watson, J. M., & Records, L. E. (1978).The effectiveness of the Porch Index of Communicative Ability as a diagnostic tool in assessing specific behaviors of senile dementia. In R. H. Brookshire (Ed.), *Clinical aphasiology conference proceedings* (pp. 93–105). Minneapolis: BRK Publishers.

Wertz, R. T. (1978). Neuropathologies of speech and language: An introduction to patient management. In D. F. Johns (Ed.), *Clinical management of neurogenic communicative disorders*. Boston: Little, Brown.

Wertz, R. T., Deal, J. L., & Robinson, A. J. (1984). Classifying the aphasias: A comparison of the Boston Diagnostic Aphasia Examination and the Western Aphasia Battery. *Clinics in Aphasiology, 14,* 164–173.

Yorkston, K. M., Beukelman. D. R., & Bell, K. R. (1988). *Clinical management of dysarthric speakers*. Boston: Little, Brown.

APPENDIX 4.A Aphasia Severity Rating Scale*

<u>APHASIA SEVERITY RATING SCALE</u>

0. No usable speech or auditory comprehension.

1. All communication is through fragmentary expression; great need for inference, questioning, and guessing by the listener. The range of information that can be exchanged is limited, and the listener carries the burden of communication.

2. Conversation about familiar subjects is possible with help from the listener. There are frequent failures to convey the idea, but patient shares the burden of communication with the examiner.

3. The patient can discuss <u>almost all everyday problems</u> with little or no assistance. Reduction of speech and/or comprehension, however, makes conversation about certain material difficult or impossible.

4. Some obvious loss of fluency in speech or facility of comprehension, without significant limitation on ideas expressed or form of expression.

5. Minimal discernible speech handicaps; patient may have subjective difficulties that are not apparent to listener.

RATING SCALE PROFILE OF SPEECH CHARACTERISTICS

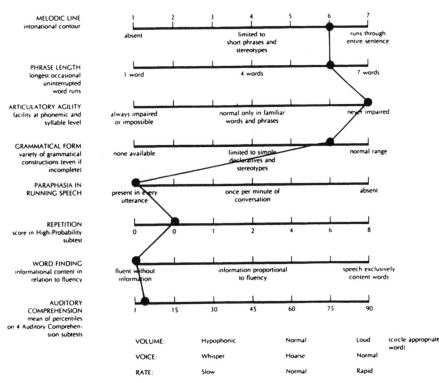

Aphasia Severity Rating Scale and rating scale profile of speech characteristics (Wernicke's aphasia) from the Boston Diagnostic Aphasia Examination.

*Reprinted with permission from H. Goodglass, & E. Kaplan, (1983). *The assessment of aphasia and related disorders* (2nd ed.) (p. 84). Philadelphia: Lea & Febiger.

APPENDIX 4.B   Aphasia Severity Rating Scale*

APHASIA SEVERITY RATING SCALE

0. No usable speech or auditory comprehension.

1. All communication is through fragmentary expression; great need for inference, questioning, and guessing by the listener. The range of information that can be exchanged is limited, and the listener carries the burden of communication.

2. Conversation about familiar subjects is possible with help from the listener. There are frequent failures to convey the idea, but patient shares the burden of communication with the examiner.

3. The patient can discuss almost all everyday problems with little or no assistance. Reduction of speech and/or comprehension, however, makes conversation about certain material difficult or impossible.

4. Some obvious loss of fluency in speech or facility of comprehension, without significant limitation on ideas expressed or form of expression.

5. Minimal discernible speech handicaps; patient may have subjective difficulties that are not apparent to listener.

RATING SCALE PROFILE OF SPEECH CHARACTERISTICS

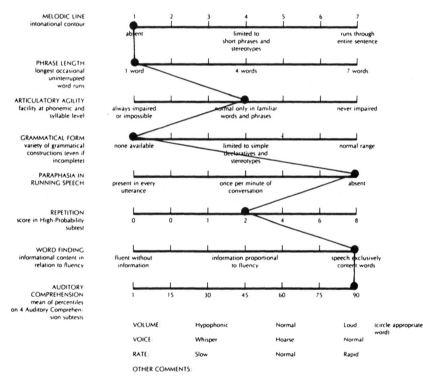

Aphasia Severity Rating Scale and rating scale profile of speech characteristics (Broca's aphasia) from the Boston Diagnostic Aphasia Examination.

---

*Reprinted with permission from H. Goodglass, & E. Kaplan, (1983). *The assessment of aphasia and related disorders* (2nd ed.) (p. 79). Philadelphia: Lea & Febiger.

5 Fluency and Voice

Tommie L. Robinson, Jr.
Thomas A. Crowe

With the number and variety of assessment options for stuttering and voice disorders increasing annually, the decision of selecting the most appropriate evaluation instrument(s) becomes increasingly more difficult for clinicians. Often clinicians select products and approaches with little more to base their decision on than name recognition or an inherited protocol. In this chapter, selected commercial and informal measures for assessing speech fluency and voice production are reviewed to assist clinicians in selecting assessment procedures appropriate to their clinical setting.

During the evaluation process for both fluency and voice, clinicians must keep in mind a number of assessment objectives:

1. Obtain ample information relative to the possible etiology and history of the disorder that facilitates differential diagnosis and prognosis.
2. Describe the disorder (dysfluency characteristics and secondary mannerisms) or vocal characteristics in clinically relevant terms.
3. Identify concomitant problems associated with stuttering or voice disorders that may influence the approach to or outcome of therapy.
4. Determine the focus of counseling (as to whether therapy is indicated, what may be realistically achieved in therapy, and so forth).
5. Understand and respond to the cultural identity of clients and their significant others.

In this chapter, commercial instruments for evaluating fluency and voice are reviewed. The theoretical construct of each instrument is presented, as well as information relative to the development, structure, and use of each instrument. A critique of the instruments reviewed follows, as well as a list of other measures and instruments.

Fluency Assessment Instruments

Evaluation of speech fluency is seen by some clinicians as one of the most challenging experiences in speech-language pathology, yet stuttering is one of the most recognized communication disorders. During the evaluation process, clinicians might find it necessary to focus on the goal of the speech fluency evaluation—that is, to obtain an adequate sample of the client's speech so that a representative sample of speech fluency and dysfluency is obtained in a variety of speaking contexts. Applying appropriate principles for gathering speech/language samples helps to facilitate skills in this area. Once this goal is met, clinicians are then faced with how to analyze the data and determine the diagnosis. Moreover, they must determine the degree to which there is an effect on the client's life as a result of the speech fluency behavior. To this end, commercial measures may be used to augment the clinical skills of the clinician and aid in the evaluation process for determining diagnosis, level of severity, and prognosis. This section describes evaluation instruments used in the area of speech fluency. Instruments of limited circulation and distribution are listed in Appendix 5A.

Evaluation Instruments Used in Speech Fluency

Cooper Personalized Fluency Control Therapy Revised

The Cooper Personalized Fluency Control Therapy Revised (PFCT-R) (E. Cooper & C. Cooper, 1985) applies to both children and adults. The assessment portion of the PFCT-R is designed to identify fluency-related attitudes and behaviors of children and adults. In addition, the perceptions of parents and teachers are assessed when evaluating children.

This program is based on the theoretical construct that "most chronic stuttering is the result of multiple coexisting physiologic and psychological factors" (E. Cooper & C. Cooper, 1985, p. 4). The authors indicate that the problem resulting from multiple coexisting factors is discoordination of the processes of phonation, articulation, and respiration.

There are several components to the kit. The handbook is divided into eight chapters and includes an assessment digest and treatment plan in two versions: children/adolescent and adult. Also included are a series of games and a black-line master booklet.

The children's evaluation is conducted by administering the PFCT-R fluency assessment digest and treatment plan. Included in the fluency assessment portion of the booklet is a chronicity prediction checklist, which includes the following assessment instruments:

- Parent assessment
- Teacher assessment
- Frequency assessment (recitation, responding, repeating, reading, picture identification, elicited spontaneous speech)
- Duration of stuttering moments
- Concomitant behaviors
- Attitudinal indicators of significance of stuttering

- Situation avoidance reactions
- Child's perceptions of severity
- Clinician's perceptions of severity

For evaluating adolescents and adults, the protocol is similar to that of the children's and includes the following assessment variables:

- Frequency of stuttering
- Duration of stuttering moments
- Situation avoidance reactions
- Concomitant behaviors
- Attitudinal indicators of significance of stuttering
- Client perceptions of severity
- Clinician perceptions of severity

For each section of the PFCT-R assessment digest, a score or percentage is assigned. After the completion of data analysis, the clinician makes a judgment as to the degree to which the disorder is handicapping, both socially and educationally, on a scale that ranges from no problem to profound involvement.

Stocker Probe for Fluency and Language
The Stocker Probe for Fluency and Language (Stocker & Goldfarb, 1995) applies to children. It is a diagnostic instrument for assessing stuttering and adult language. According to Stocker and Goldfarb (1995), the Stocker Probe technique is based on the notion that breakdowns in speech fluency occur as a result of increased speech demands. This model is based on the demands-capacities model (Starkweather, 1987; Starkweather et al., 1990). The assessment instrument is divided into two parts: Part I is the Stocker Probe for Fluency, and part II is the Stocker Probe for Language.

The fluency portion is addressed in five steps. During the initial step, several events take place. First, the administration of the "I" (initial) probes is presented. According to Stocker and Goldfarb (1995), "a probe consists of a series of questions or requests about two different common objects presented to the child" (p. 15). The questions or requests are presented in random order and build on a hierarchy relative to the level of demands on the speaker.

A level I question involves the use of an "either/or question," in which the answer is implicit in the question and is a low-level expressive language task. The idea is to elicit a short repetition response. For example, the clinician gives the child a ball and asks, "Is it old or new?"

A level II question is similar to a level I in that it elicits a short response, but it requires the child to name a common object. However, the name of the object is not given in the question (for example, "What is it?").

A level III question elicits a response usually consisting of a prepositional phrase in which the referents are not present or named in the question (for example, "Where would you keep one?").

Level IV involves eliciting a series of attributes also not part of the request. "Tell me everything you know about it" is the task that is presented to the child, for example. The child is expected to demonstrate the use of expanded sentences. In this level, unlike levels II and III, the child's response is not constrained by the nature of the question.

Level V is the highest level of the probe. The child is asked to participate in a narrative discourse task. According to the authors, this is the most creative task of the probe and often elicits the most complex response. During the administration of this probe, each of the levels is administered twice, making a total of 10 demands per evaluation. A random order is used to give the child an opportunity to recover fluency if there were dysfluent moments during administration of the first series.

For scoring, clinicians are encouraged to audiotape or videotape the session. All scoring is either [+] or [–] on the Stocker Probe recording sheet that accompanies the program. The [+] is used for fluent responses, and the [–] is used for dysfluent responses. The amount and type of dysfluency are not recorded on any level but are noted. A response is considered to be dysfluent as soon as the dysfluency occurs. Clinicians are to wait until an entire fluent response is completed before determining a score for the response. During the evaluation process, five probes with 10 responses for each are administered (for a total of 50). A severity rating scale is provided. This evaluation system is used also for ongoing or weekly probes. However, there are only 10 responses and two presentations for each level.

Stuttering Prediction Instrument for Young Children

The Stuttering Prediction Instrument for Young Children (Riley, 1981) was developed to provide speech-language pathologists with assessment data when dealing with complex decisions that are often associated with stuttering. There is a need for an instrument that answers some of the complex questions that arise when working with a child who stutters. A set of six criteria was created by Riley (1981) to foster the development of this instrument:

1. It should be simple enough for routine clinical use by observed trainers.
2. It should quantify behaviors that are consistently identified as abnormal dysfluencies and assign weights to them compatible with experienced clinical judgment and, when possible, research findings.
3. It should have appropriate reliability and validity characteristics to meet American Psychological Association standards.
4. It should be standardized on a large representative sample of children who stutter and a control group of children who do not stutter.
5. It should yield data useful in developing and monitoring treatment goals.
6. It should have predictive validity to justify longitudinal studies.

Administration of the instrument involves three procedures. The first obtains information regarding the child who stutters through background information, family history of stuttering, and reactions of parents/caregivers to the stuttering. The second observes two dysfluency types (part-word repetitions and prolongations) and their frequencies for any signs of abnormality. The clinician also obtains a language sample of at least 100 words by engaging the child in conversation to observe associated behaviors—that is, phonatory arrest and articulatory posturing. The third completes an analysis of the tape-recorded language sample.

Scoring is carried out by conducting an analysis of the tape-recorded sample. A dot [.] is used to identify each fluent word and a diagonal line [/] for each stuttered word. A minimum of 100 words is needed to complete the task. The number of stuttering events is divided by the number of words analyzed and the total multiplied by 100 for a percentage of words stuttered. This percentage is then converted to a score and is added to the other sections to determine a total score out of a possible range of 0 to 40. The author also provides results of reliability and validity studies and information regarding predicting chronicity.

Materials needed during the administration of this tool are the test form, a tape recorder, and a copy of the manual. Included in the manual is a list of topics to elicit conversation and a series of picture plates.

Stuttering Severity Instrument for Children and Adults (3rd ed.)

The development of the Stuttering Severity Instrument for Children and Adults (3rd ed.; Riley, 1994) was based on the following criteria:

1. It must be simple enough to be used by a trained clinician in any reasonable clinical setting.
2. It must be as objective as possible. The behaviors to be judged must be externally visible or audible.
3. It must be sensitive enough to register changes in severity that are clinically significant, even if the differences are not readily apparent to the untrained observer.
4. The psychometric characteristics (reliability and validity) must be acceptable for clinic and research use.
5. Normative data must be available so that a given sample of stuttering can be evaluated on a standardized scale.
6. The instrument should be usable for both children and adults.

The instrument is based on three parameters that were the basis for the original Stuttering Severity Instrument (Riley, 1972) and well as the revised Stuttering Severity Instrument (Riley, 1980). These parameters include

1. Frequency of repetitions and prolongations of sounds and syllables
2. Estimated duration of the longest stuttering events
3. Observable physical concomitant behaviors

The current edition allows clinicians or researchers to select additional parameters, such as word or situation avoidance, percentage of stuttered words or syllables, speech rate, average duration of stuttering, and other relevant variables. Clinicians use the test form and need to audio- or videotape the procedure.

The Stuttering Severity Instrument test record and frequency computation form is divided into four major sections: *frequency* (converted to scaled scores 0–18); *duration* (converted to scaled scores 0–18); *physical concomitants* (rated by degree of distractibility 0–20); and *severity conversion tables* for preschool children (ages 2 years, 10 months to 5 years, 11 months), school-age children (ages 6 years, 0 months to 16 years, 11 months), and adults (ages 17 years, 0 months and older). Each table expresses the score as a stanine equivalent and suggests a descriptive severity level (very mild, mild, moderate, etc.). Alternative methods for counting dysfluencies are allowed, and stimulus materials are included with the test.

The author provides guidelines for administering the instrument, and it can be used with nonreaders and readers. For nonreaders, the following scores are computed: frequency, duration, physical concomitants, and total overall. Children and adults who can read are administered the speaking tasks (familiar topic) as well as a reading task on the appropriate grade level.

Scores calculated for each section, and a total overall score, percentile rank, and severity levels are provided. Interpretation of the test results is based on normative data provided for each of the three age levels.

The author provides intraexaminer and interexaminer reliability for each of the areas assessed and reports reliability figures ranging from 82% to 93%. Criterion-related and construct validity were also addressed and psychometric data presented.

Assessment of Fluency in School-Age Children

The Assessment of Fluency in School-Age Children (Thompson, 1983) applies to children aged 6–17 years. It is a criterion-referenced instrument that is used to provide clinicians with identification, referral, evaluation, therapy, and dismissal information. This instrument is based on the differential evaluation framework developed by Gregory (1973) and the evaluation process developed by Williams et al. (1978). Gregory (1979) suggests that there are different types of stutterers, different avenues to becoming a stutterer, or contributing factors which combine in various ways to produce stuttering. Williams et al. (1978) recommend a procedure that explores a variety of different avenues for addressing stuttering in school-age children. These include obtaining a case history, teacher profiles, attitude surveys, and taped samples of conversation and reading. Additionally, they suggest that a comprehensive examination include listeners' and speakers' reactions and attitudes and the speech behavior of the speaker.

The assessment kit contains several items that are important to the evaluation process: the parent interview form, teacher evaluation form, resource guide, and assessment record form. Additional diagnostic test materials include a tape recorder, stopwatch, crayons, blank paper, sequence pictures, picture storybook, and screening tests for articulation and syntax.

The assessment record form is used to record information such as

1. *Automatic speech*: The child is asked to count to 40, name the days of the week, or recite the alphabet. This activity is used to determine efficient use of exhaled air.
2. *Cued speech*: The student names pictures, repeats sentences, tells a story using sequence cards, and describes a picture from a storybook. Fluency is monitored, and the results recorded.

3. *Spontaneous speech*: The student is instructed to choose a topic for presentation (monologue), engage in dialogue, and discuss a picture that he or she draws.
4. *Physiologic components*: An oral motor assessment is made, and breathing is assessed.
5. *Interview with student*: Attitudes are elicited for assessment.

There is an optional portion of the evaluation in which fluency disrupters are used while the child engages in dialogue. During the evaluation, language and speech components are rated, and a 100- to 150-word representative sample of the child's speech is transcribed and rated for speech fluency. The types of dysfluencies are rated using a list of codes, and the number of speech dysfluencies is divided by the total number of words spoken in the transcript. The number is multiplied by 100 to determine a percentage.

Assessment and Therapy Programme for Dysfluent Children

The Assessment and Therapy Programme for Dysfluent Children (Rustin, 1987) is designed to provide intervention goals. Requisite to intervention is a complete assessment and an in-depth understanding of the family's lifestyle. The parents are considered an important part of the assessment, and both are required for an interview before interaction with the child. The theoretical focus of this program is pragmatic in nature and is based on different etiologies of stuttering. Theoretical positions include works by Jonas (1977), who suggested an eclectic point of view as to the cause of stuttering; Curlee and Perkins (1984), who linked stuttering to operant behavior, prosody, cognition, linguistics, sequencing, timing, and temporal programming; Cooper (1976) and Gregory (1986), who suggested a correlation to physiologic, psychological, genetic, and environmental variables; Moore and Boberg (1987), who presented information relative to central nervous system involvement; Moore and Haynes (1980), who emphasized right hemisphere involvement; Andrews et al. (1983), who articulated a relationship with speech and language development; and Peters (1986), who linked speech motor behavior to stuttering.

The assessment procedure includes a parent interview and interaction with the child. There are guidelines for asking questions. Suggested topics are

1. *Present complaint*: The clinician asks, "What is the nature of the problem?"
2. *Detailed description of stuttering*: Parents are asked to describe and give examples of the dysfluent behavior.
3. *Recent behavior and emotional state*: This section contains questions regarding general health, eating, sleeping and elimination, muscular system and concentration, speech, tics and mannerisms, attachment disorders, emotions, peer relationships, relationships with siblings, relationships with adults, antisocial trends, sex education, and schooling.
4. *Family structure and history*: According to the author, this section is referred to as "the core of the interview procedure, and deals with personal details of the parents' lives" (Rustin, 1987, p. 7). It has ques-

tions pertaining to marriage, history of previous pregnancies, personal background, description of parent's personality, emotional problems, parents' family backgrounds, and extended family issues.

5. *Family life and relationships*: This section is an assessment of the actual home environment. It includes topics such as parental relationships, parent-child interaction, child's participation in family activities, family pattern of relationships, and discipline.

6. *Child's development history*: This portion of the test focuses on the development of motor milestones as well as the mother/child relationship.

7. *Temperamental or personality attributes*: This section explores the child's adaptation to a variety of situations and gives attention to motivation.

During the final portion of the parent interview, the clinician shares with the parents some general information and a short overview of facts known about stuttering. Information that guides the discussion of the clinician and parents is provided in the child assessment booklet.

The aims of the child assessment are to

- Assess the amount and types of dysfluency present
- Explore the child's attitudes and feelings
- Experiment with various ways of modifying the child's stuttering behavior
- Identify associated problems

Materials needed for the assessment include

1. Child assessment booklet
2. Stopwatch
3. Tally counter
4. Tape recorder
5. Reading materials
6. Ten easily identified, single-object pictures
7. Calculator

Speech samples are elicited in a variety of speaking situations that include automatic speech, echoic speech, reading, naming pictures, monologue, responding to questions, and conversational sample. For each of these tasks, a representative sample of the child's speech is obtained.

After the speech samples are elicited, number of words spoken for each section and the figures for time, stuttered words, and words spoken are totaled. The totaled time in seconds is converted to minutes and seconds. In addition, the types of stuttered words are identified. Finally, the stuttered words per minute, percentage of stuttered words, and words spoken per minute are calculated.

The final stage of the assessment is the child interview, in which the child's attitudes and feelings are explored. The clinician is instructed to ask open-ended questions relative to school, home, and speech.

Crowe's Protocols: A Comprehensive Guide to Stuttering Assessment

Crowe's Protocols (Crowe et al., 2000) applies to children and adults. This evaluation tool provides a comprehensive assessment of stuttering and the person who stutters. It addresses all dimensions of stuttering—"the sound, look, and feel" of stuttering—for both the child client and the adult client. General features of Crowe's Protocols include

1. *Counseling relevance*: Sections and forms are designed to provide information that may prove useful in informative and personal adjustment counseling at various stages of the evaluation and treatment processes.
2. *Cultural assessment*: A section is provided to assist the clinician in determining the relevance of the client's culture to his or her reactions to stuttering. This information is intended for use in counseling and in structuring therapy.
3. *Protocols*: This section is structured to provide a composite, comprehensive profile of the client's stuttering and his or her reactions to it. The sections and forms chosen to be administered may vary among clients. The sections also can be prioritized differently for each client and administered over time.
4. *Abbreviated protocol*: An abbreviated protocol is suggested (in an appendix) for clinicians with limited time for initial evaluation sessions.
5. *Cross-referencing forms*: Forms are cross-referencing in order to provide a composite assessment of the client's stuttering and to facilitate determination of stuttering severity, differential diagnosis, prognosis, and therapy planning.
6. *Scaling of assessment results*: The client characteristics forms in Crowe's Protocols are constructed with 3-point and 7-point scales. Summary scales are provided for an overall rating of each characteristic assessed. The scaled forms are intended to enable the clinician to establish baselines for various features of the client's stuttering, document change across time in the client's stuttering, and document the outcomes of therapy. The scaled forms are also intended to aid in determining the severity of a client's stuttering and prognosis for therapy.

Crowe's Protocols contains the following sections and forms:

1. *Case history*: General information, description of the problem, history of the problem, family/environmental information, medical history
2. *Cultural factors*
3. *Client assessment*

The client assessment section breaks down further into

1. *General assessment*: Client questionnaire, school questionnaire, perceptions of stuttering, speech and fluency demands
2. *Affective assessment*: Emotional responses to stuttering, attitudes toward stuttering, self-image

3. *Behavioral assessment*: Conversational sample, transcription form, frequency and type of dysfluency, location of dysfluencies, duration of dysfluencies, phonetic type, latency of response, length of response, reading samples, reading passages, consistency of dysfluencies, accompanying physical behaviors
4. *Cognitive assessment*: Cognitive indicators of stuttering severity, situational ratings, avoidance behaviors, speech locus of control
5. *General speech status*: Communicative effectiveness, communicative naturalness, degree of handicap
6. *Stimulability*: Stimulability, stimulability reading passages
7. *Severity*: severity of stuttering, severity of stuttering progress form

The forms are designed to be completed by the client or by the clinician through respondent interview. Reading passages are provided for use in behavioral assessment of the client's stuttering and in stimulability assessment.

Critique of Speech Fluency Instruments

Positive Aspects

In light of the fact that stuttering remains one of the most abstruse speech disorders to evaluate and treat, the authors of the various diagnostic instruments reviewed here have developed helpful protocols and strategies for evaluating children and adults who stutter. Their products represent extensive research and clinical trials on their part to develop instruments that address the causes and correlates of stuttering.

It is to be noted that numerous researchers have emphasized the significance of the role that parents play in shaping their children's fluency development and in the stuttering intervention process. This opinion is reflected in several of the instruments reviewed in this chapter (i.e., Cooper & Cooper, 1985; Riley, 1981; Rustin, 1987; Thompson, 1983). The authors of these instruments suggest that it is important to include parents in the clinical interaction as their child's speech fluency is analyzed and to rely on them as historians/reporters of the child's environmental, medical, social, developmental, and emotional histories.

The involvement of teachers in the stuttering intervention process is also addressed in several of the evaluation instruments reviewed here (Cooper & Cooper, 1985; Thompson, 1983). This aspect of interaction is important to the overall management of children and adolescents. Because children and adolescents who stutter spend a relatively large amount of time in schools—interacting with their teachers, classmates, and peers as well as, in some cases, experiencing stress, communication pressure, and social isolation—assessment of the school environment and the teacher-student relationship is critical. Information directly related to the school dynamic can be factored into the development of goals and objectives for the treatment process.

The instruments reviewed here also rely on supplemental information that is gathered in addition to the regular diagnostic data. For example, the authors encourage the clinicians to use audio- and videotape as mechanisms for further monitoring of dysfluency and associated behaviors. This is not only useful for an initial counting and typing of dysfluencies, but also for reliability checks of clinician skills and for monitoring the progress of intervention across time.

Limiting Aspects

Each of the instruments reviewed in this chapter fails to address the need to consider multicultural issues in evaluation of stuttering. Cultural adjustments can be made, however, to most programs if judged necessary by the clinician. Robinson and Crowe (1998) provide a paradigm for addressing cultural factors when providing services to multicultural populations. These suggestions can be incorporated into the diagnostic process as needed by clinicians.

Another area not addressed by some of the evaluation instruments reviewed is identification of types of dysfluencies during the client's dysfluent moments. These instruments provide instructions for recognizing and recording dysfluent moments, but not for recognizing the type of dysfluency. Using the [.] and [/]—as in the Stuttering Prediction Instrument and the Stuttering Severity Instrument (Riley, 1981, 1994)—is brief, quick, and can be done with accuracy; however, this current system does not allow the clinician to distinguish a block from a prolongation. Clinicians may find that developing an abbreviation system for determining the type of dysfluency may aid in addressing this concern.

There is much discussion of the need for outcomes data in today's clinical environment. It is important that evaluation instruments offer baseline data for comparison during and after treatment. With changes in health care and service delivery in the schools, clinicians are required to document and provide evidence of improvement during the course of treatment. The initial step for addressing treatment outcomes is a thorough data-driven evaluation. Although this has not been addressed formally within the evaluation programs presented here, these evaluation instruments can in fact become the initial step in a process for establishing a protocol to monitor the outcomes of therapy.

Other Fluency Assessment Measures

Curlee and Perkins (1984) provide calculations for the measurement of stuttering moments. They include

1. *Percent of syllables stuttered*: This is determined by taking the total number of stutterings and dividing it by the total number of syllables spoken. This number is then multiplied by 100.
2. *Average duration of stutterings*: Ten representative stuttering moments (relative to length) are randomly selected. The sum of the total time is divided by 10 to determine the average.
3. *Duration of the three longest stutterings*: Using a stopwatch, the three longest stutterings in a speech sample are timed.
4. *Overall speaking rate (approximate) calculated in syllables per minute*: This is determined by taking the number of syllables spoken in a 2-minute speaking sample and dividing by the number 2.

5. *Articulatory rate*: To determine the average articulatory rate or average syllables per minute, the total number of nonstuttered syllables should be divided by the total amount of talk time.

6. *Average duration of nonstuttered intervals*: To compute this number, the clinicians should determine the total amount of nonstuttered talking time and divide it by the number of actual nonstuttered utterances.

7. *Duration of the three longest nonstuttered intervals*: The clinician must judge what he or she considers to be the three longest periods of speaking without stuttering. The time (in minutes and seconds) should be recorded on the stuttering data sheet.

8. *Average length of nonstuttered intervals*: The number is computed by collecting the total number of nonstuttered syllables and dividing it by the actual number of utterances measured. The authors suggested using 10 utterances, but more can be used.

9. *Length of the three longest nonstuttered intervals*: Using the stuttering rating data sheet, clinicians are encouraged to observe the longest nonstuttered interval in a sample and count the number of syllables emitted. These three numbers are recorded on the form.

10. *Naturalness rating*: The authors provide a stuttering rating data sheet using a 9-point scale (1 = highly natural; 0 = highly unnatural) that may be used with laypeople or clients.

Culatta and Goldberg (1995) identified an assessment variable that they refer to as the perceived severity of stuttering. They indicate that both visual and auditory features of stuttering influence clients as well as listeners in judging severity of stutterings. Based on the work of Martin et al. (1984), perceived severity of stuttering is a rating of "natural and unnatural" speech to the degree of deviancy. Williams et al. (1978) developed a scale of rating severity of stuttering that is used for this assessment.

Voice Assessment Instruments

Evaluation of voice often is viewed by clinicians as being a process defined by dichotomous orientations: instrumentation-based versus perceptual, objective versus subjective, and medical versus nonmedical. Ideally, choice among these orientations is unnecessary at the time of evaluation. Ideally, the clinician has access to and experience with equipment designed for laryngeal examination and voice analysis, an ear finely tuned to the parameters of voice, skill in using objective (that is not necessary to say instrumentation) measures of voice, the skill and confidence to make subjective judgments, and access to and working relationship with medical professionals who are experienced with voice and pathologies that adversely affect voice. Yet even with the support of instrumentation-based voice/laryngeal analysis and medical consultation, the clinician may find that he or she relies most heavily on subjective-perceptual methods for voice evaluation. In the information that follows, a review of current voice assessment instruments is provided. Voice assessment instruments with limited circulation and distribution are listed in Appendix 5B.

Voice Assessment Protocol for Children and Adults

The Voice Assessment Protocol for Children and Adults (VAP; Pindzola, 1997) is a voice assessment instrument that is appropriate for both children and adults. The VAP assesses the voice parameters of pitch, loudness, quality, breath features, and rate/rhythm. Instrumentation is not necessary to use the protocol.

Materials necessary to conduct the evaluation include a pencil, tape recorder, stopwatch, and appropriate auditory perceptual skills. Clinicians are advised to enhance perceptual judgment by using a variety of low- and high-technology instrumentation, such as musical instrument(s), pitch pipe, sound spectrograph, and loudness indicator. The different subtests are as follows:

1. *Pitch assessment*: The author provides helpful guidance for establishing pitch, pitch variability, diplophonia, and pitch breaks. An appendix that contains activities to aid in determining the habitual pitch of the client is included.
2. *Loudness assessment*: This subtest of the VAP furnishes information about loudness level, degree of effort, loudness consistency, articulatory impact, and daily vocal use. The protocol allows clinicians to record information on the form, and space is available for making supplemental notes.
3. *Quality assessment*: The clinician judges quality according to the parameters of breathiness, harshness, or hoarseness. The clinician is also urged to mark tonal deviations using the categories severe and distracting; moderate in degree; slight or intermittent; or not present, normal. Glottal approximation and resonance problems are also identified in this section.
4. *Breath features*: The author indicates that breathing variables are important to vocal loudness and rate of speech. Information regarding predominate region of breathing, sounds associated with breathing for speech, average number of words per breath group, maximum duration of /a/ and S/Z ratio is obtained.
5. *Rate and rhythm*: Rate of speech is quantified during the conversation. Number of words per minute and number of syllables per minute are calculated, and diadochokinesis determined.

The author indicates that an appropriate speech sample and a well-trained ear are needed to complete the protocol. Included with this assessment is an audiotape that includes different pitch level samples.

Boone Voice Program for Children (2nd ed.)

The Boone Voice Program for Children (Boone, 1993) is designed to assess the voice characteristics of children and includes screening and in-depth protocols. The evaluation is completed before referral to the physician. This program provides step-by-step guidelines and materials for the diagnostic and remediation processes. The program consists of the following components: (1) an instruction manual for screening, evaluation, and referral; (2) voice evaluation forms; (3) voice report for parents forms; (4) voice referral to physician forms; and (5) a cassette for ear training and establishing new pitch.

The voice evaluation form consists of ten sections that encompass history of the voice problem, health history, hearing evaluation, oral peripheral evaluation, nasal resonance evaluation, respiration evaluation, phonation evaluation, voice rating scale, observations, and summary and plan:

1. *History of the voice problem*: The clinician records the identifying information and obtains the description of the problem, cause of the problem, and onset of the problem. In addition, questions are posed regarding prior therapy, voice variability throughout the day, and overall voice usage.

2. *Health history*: This section is designed to provide an overall medical/health history. Such information includes birth history, feeding problems, illnesses and allergies, and medication.

3. *Hearing evaluation*: A pure-tone audiometric screening or threshold screening is completed. The child's ability to discriminate pitch and his or her tonal memory are also assessed in this section.

4. *Oral peripheral evaluation*: A peripheral speech mechanism examination and diadochokinetic rates are elicited for the purpose of examining structure and function.

5. *Nasal resonance evaluation*: Resonance balance is judged both during the assessment and with specific materials.

6. *Respiration evaluation*: Assessment of respiration is a very important portion of the evaluation. A checklist is provided, along with information for measuring vital capacity and total capacity. The S/Z ratio is also computed.

7. *Phonation evaluation*: This section requires some form of instrumentation to complete the laryngoscopic/endoscopic/stroboscopic exam. Each of the techniques provides different information. The endoscopic exam can provide helpful videotape information that shows supraglottal structures during phonation. The stroboscopic exam shows the motion of the vocal folds and enables the clinician to see details such as vocal fold approximation and closure, mucosal edge, mucosal wave, and whether the vocal folds seem to come together and vibrate at the same time. Additional information regarding perturbation values, pitch evaluation, pitch range, natural pitch, and habitual pitch can be collected with the appropriate instrumentation.

8. *Voice rating scale*: A voice rating scale assesses the voice parameters of breathing, loudness, pitch, pitch inflections, quality, horizontal focus, vertical focus, and nasal resonance.

9. *Observations*: Behavioral information is recorded in this section. Areas of concern may include such features as eye contact, postural behavior, and vocal abuse behavior.

10. *Summary and plan*: The final section is used to summarize the clinician's assessment data and plan for managing behavior.

After the clinician completes the evaluation process, it may be necessary to refer for a medical examination. The author provides a form for this task. In addition, a voice report form for parents is included as part of the materials.

Critique of Voice Instruments

Positive Aspects

In contrast with fluency assessment instruments, there is a limited number of diagnostic protocols to examine vocal quality subjectively. Researchers have reported that the best voice assessment instrument is a well-trained ear. The authors of the instruments reviewed in this chapter do an excellent job of presenting frameworks for perceptual assessment of voice. Another added feature of these assessment tools is that they allow for the use of instrumentation to enhance the quality of the evaluation (for example, musical instrument[s], pitch pipe, and sound spectrography) and to supplement perceptual judgment.

Limiting Aspects

In line with the comments regarding the fluency instruments reviewed, it can be indicated that the influence of culture on vocal characteristics is not addressed by the instruments reviewed herein. Researchers indicate that cultural factors affect the quality of the voice and may be reflected in all of the parameters of the voice. DeJarnette and Holland (1993, 1998) offer a number of suggestions for the prevention and assessment of voice disorders in multicultural populations using ethnographic information relative to anatomic, physiologic, acoustic, perceptual, cultural, and linguistic parameters.

There is a need for researchers and clinicians to link the voice evaluation process to treatment outcomes. As with the fluency evaluation process, this is a particularly critical issue in terms of clinical accountability and reimbursement issues.

References

Andrews, G., Craig, A., Feyer, A. M., Hoddinott, S., Howie, P., & Neilson, M. (1983). Stuttering: A review of research, findings and theories. *Journal of Speech and Hearing Disorders, 48,* 226–246.

Boone, D. R. (1993). *The Boone voice program for children* (2nd ed.). Austin, TX: Pro-Ed.

Cooper, E. G. (1976). *Personalized fluency control therapy: An integrated behavior and relationship therapy for stutterers.* Austin, TX: Learning Concepts.

Cooper, E., & Cooper, C. (1985). *Cooper personalized fluency control therapy (revised).* Austin, TX: Pro-Ed.

Crowe, A., Di Lollo, A., & Bradley, T. (2000). *Crowe's protocols: A comprehensive guide to stuttering assessment.* San Antonio, TX: Psychological Corporation.

Culatta, R., & Goldberg, S. A. (1995). *Stuttering therapy: An integrated approach to theory and practice.* Needham Heights, MA: Allyn & Bacon.

Curlee, R. F., & Perkins, W. H. (Eds). (1984). *Nature and treatment of stuttering: New directions.* San Diego: College Hill Press.

DeJarnette, G., & Holland, R. W. (1993). Voice and voice disorders. In D. Battle (Ed.), *Communication disorders in multicultural populations* (pp. 212–238). Boston: Andover Medical Publishers.

DeJarnette, G., & Holland, R. W. (1998). Voice and voice disorders. In D. Battle (Ed.), *Communication disorders in multicultural populations* (2nd ed) (pp. 257–307). Boston: Andover Medical Publishers.

Gregory, H. (1973). *Stuttering: An introduction to differential evaluation and therapy.* Indianapolis: Bobbs-Merrill Company, Inc.

Gregory, H. (1979). *Controversies about stuttering therapy.* Baltimore: University Park Press.

Gregory, H. (1986). *Stuttering: Differential evaluation and therapy.* Austin, TX: Pro-Ed.

Jonas, G. (1977). *Stuttering: The disorders of many theories.* New York: Farrar, Strauss and Giroux.

Martin, R.R., Haroldson, S.K., & Trident, K.A. (1984). Stuttering and speech naturalness. *Journal of Speech and Hearing Research, 49,* 53–58.

Moore, W. H., & Boberg, E. (1987). Hermispheric processing and stuttering. In L. Rustin, D. Rowley & H. Purser (Eds.). *Progress in the treatment of fluency disorders* (pp. 19–42). London: Taylor Francis.

Moore, W. H., & Haynes, W. O. (1980). Alpha hemispheric asymmetry and stuttering: Some support for a segmentation disfunction hypothesis. *Journal of Speech and Hearing Research, 23,* 292–297.

Peters, H. F. (1986). Limitations and possibilities in speech motor behaviour in stuttering. Presented the International Symposium on Physiology and Therapy in Stuttering: Brussels.

Pindzola, R. H., & White, D. T. (1986). A protocol for differentiating the incipient stutterer. *Language, Speech, and Hearing Services in the Schools, 17,* 12–15.

Riley, G. D. (1972). A stuttering severity instrument for children and adults. *Journal of Speech and Hearing Disorders, 37,* 314–320.

Riley, G. (1980). *Stuttering severity instrument for children and adults (revised).* Austin, TX: Pro-Ed.

Riley, G. (1981). *Stuttering prediction instrument for young children.* Austin, TX: Pro-Ed.

Riley, G. (1994). *Stuttering severity instrument for children* (3rd ed.). Austin, TX: Pro-Ed.

Robinson, T. L. Jr., & Crowe, T. A. (1998). Culture-based considerations in programming for stuttering intervention in African American clients and their families. *Language, Speech, and Hearing Services in the Schools, 29,* 172–179.

Rustin, L. (1987). *Assessment and therapy programme for dysfluent children.* Tucson, AZ: Communication Skill Builders, Inc.

Starkweather, C. W. (1987). *Fluency and stuttering*. Englewood Cliffs, NJ: Prentice-Hall.

Starkweather, C. W., Gottwald, S. R., & Halfond, M. M. (1990). *Stuttering prevention: A clinical method*. Englewood Cliffs, NJ: Prentice-Hall.

Stocker, B., & Goldfarb, R. (1995). *The Stocker probe for fluency and language*. Vero Beach, FL: The Speech Bin.

Thompson, J. (1983). *Assessment of fluency in school-age children*. Austin, TX: Pro-Ed.

Williams, D. E., Darley, F. L., & Spriestersbach, D. C. (1978). Differential diagnosis of disorders of fluency. In F. L. Darley & D. C. Spriestersbach (Eds.), *Diagnostic methods in speech pathology* (2nd ed.) (pp. 409–438). New York: Harper & Row.

APPENDIX 5.A   Other Speech Fluency Assessment Instruments

Iowa Scale of Attitude Toward Stuttering

Ammons, R. B., & Johnson, W. (1963). Iowa scale of attitude toward stuttering. In W. Johnson, F. L. Darley, & D. C. Spristersbach (Eds.), *Diagnostic methods in speech pathology* (pp. 39–49). New York: Harper & Row.

Stuttering Diagnostic and Evaluation Checklist

Luper, H. I., & Mulder, R. I. (1966). *Stuttering therapy for children.* Englewood Cliffs, NJ: Prentice-Hall.

Perceptions of Stuttering Inventory

Woolf, G. (1967). Perceptions of stuttering inventory. *British Journal of Disorders of Communication, 2,* 158–177.

Stuttering Severity Scale

Lanyon, R. I. (1967). The measurement of stuttering severity. *Journal of Speech and Hearing Research, 10,* 836–843.

Measures of Dysfluency of Speaking and Oral Reading

Williams, D. E., Darley, F. L., & Spriestersbach, D. C. (1978). Differential diagnosis of disorders of fluency. In F. L. Darley & D. C. Spriestersbach (Eds.), *Diagnostic methods in speech pathology* (2nd ed.) (pp. 409–438). New York: Harper & Row.

Checklist of Stuttering Behavior

See Williams et al. (1978).

Stutterers Self-Ratings of Reactions to Speech Situations

See Williams et al. (1978).

Scale for Rating Severity of Stuttering

See Williams et al. (1978).

Systematic Fluency Training Assessment Form

Shine, R. E. (1980). *Systematic fluency training for children.* Tigard, OR: C.C. Publications.

Stuttering Problem Profile

Silverman, F. (1980). The stuttering problem profile: A task that assists both client and clinician in defining therapy goals. *Journal of Speech and Hearing Disorders, 45,* 119–123.

Child Fluency Assessment Instrument

Goldberg, S. A. (1981). *Behavioral cognitive stuttering therapy (BCST): The rapid development of fluent speech.* Tigard, OR: C.C. Publications.

Adolescent Fluency Assessment Instrument

See Goldberg (1981).

Adult Fluency Assessment Instrument

See Goldberg (1981).

The Preschool Fluency Development Program: Assessment and Treatment

Culp, D. M. (1984). The preschool fluency development program: Assessment and treatment. In M. Peins (Ed.), *Contemporary approaches to stuttering therapy* (pp. 39–71). Boston: Little, Brown & Company, 39–71.

Protocol for Differentiating the Incipient Stutterer

Pindzola, R. H., & White, D. T. (1986). A protocol for differentiating the incipient stutterer. *Language, Speech, and Hearing Services in the Schools, 17,* 12–15.

Stuttering Assessment Protocol

Culatta, R., & Goldberg, S. A. (1995). *Stuttering therapy: An integrated approach to theory and practice*. Needham Heights, MA: Allyn & Bacon.

APPENDIX 5.B   Other Voice Assessment Measures

Wilson Voice Profile

Wilson, F. B., & Rice, M. (1977). *A programmed approach to voice therapy.* Allen, TX: DLM Teaching Resources.

Buffalo III Speech Voice Profile System

Wilson, D. K, (1987). *Voice problems in children* (3rd ed.). Baltimore: Williams & Wilkins.

6   Examination of the Oral Mechanism

Dennis M. Ruscello

An examination of the oral mechanism is generally carried out during most communicative and behavioral feeding assessments. The purpose is to identify differences in anatomy and physiology that may adversely affect communication or related functions (St. Louis & Ruscello, 2000) — that is, the practitioner needs to detect the problem and determine if there is some impact. In some cases, it is also necessary to refer clients to other disciplines when variations are noted. For example, an observed alignment problem of the upper and lower jaws may require referral to an orthodontist for examination and treatment, if necessary. In other cases, structural or physiologic variations may not adversely affect the client, but identification of the problem assists the practitioner in treating the individual. An example is a young school-aged child who exhibits a lisp in the presence of missing upper front teeth. Knowledge of dental and phonological development would be important in understanding the problem and providing both an accurate assessment and recommendations to delay management. However, the practitioners must also be mindful of the fact that there is a wide range in what is considered normal in structure and function of the oral mechanism; consequently, causal relationships cannot always be established between observable anatomic or physiologic deficits and speech or related functions such as deglutition.

In this chapter, the functional components of the oral examination are discussed, as well as differences that may be present. In addition, there are formalized tests that may be used for this purpose, and they are reviewed for the reader. Finally, there are other data and literature that may be used in conducting an examination of the speech mechanism; this information is included in the appendices for potential use.

Oral Examination

Preparation

The client must be positioned correctly to view the oral anatomy. Preferably, the client should be seated in a comfortable chair that enables an unobstructed view of the entire face. The head and trunk should be at a 90-degree angle to the lower body. The head should be straight and not in an extended or downward position. If the recommended positioning cannot be achieved because of some physical disability, the most comfortable position for the client should be achieved.

The practitioner should be seated in front and slightly to the side of the client. It may be necessary during the course of the examination for the examiner to change his or her position so that the appropriate observations can be made. The practitioner also needs to be cognizant of the fact that some clients are apprehensive of an oral examination, whereas others may be defensive to tactile stimulation and resist oral observation and contact. Because of these potential problems, it may be necessary in some cases to postpone or refrain from conducting certain portions of an oral examination. Figures 6.1 and 6.2 show clients who are preparing to undergo oral mechanism examinations.

The typical materials used in conducting the examination include tongue blades, a light source, and tissues. A stopwatch or other instru-

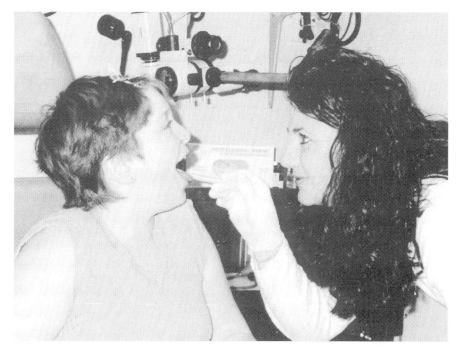

FIGURE 6.1 *The clinician obtains information relative to the structure and function of the client's oral mechanism.*

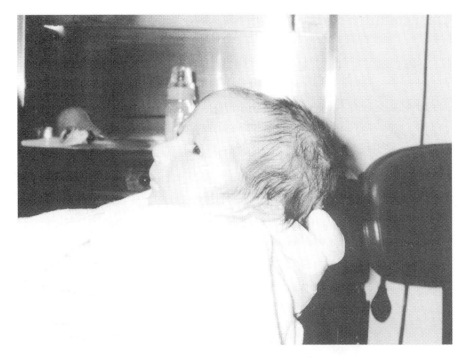

FIGURE 6.2 *The client is preparing to undergo an oral mechanism examination.*

mentation may also be used to collect performance data on speech and nonspeech oral mechanism tasks. Infection control is a concern that should be an important priority because of person-to-person contact. Rubber gloves should be worn at all times, and practitioners should wash their hands before and after administering an oral examination (McMillan & Willette, 1988). Additional safeguards must be taken in special cases. Practitioners should refer to publications regarding infection control that have been prepared by the American Speech-Language Hearing Association Committee on Quality Assurance (ASHA, 1991b; ASHA, 1990).

Conducting an Examination of the Oral Mechanism

Before conducting an examination, the practitioner should inspect the face to determine if there are any unusual facial features. It is possible that observed differences are part of a morphologic problem that also has an effect on speech production skills. Coston and his associates (1992) have developed a screening instrument that may be used to identify facial features that appear anomalous. A reproduction of the screening instrument is included in this chapter (Appendix 6A). In addition to the screening instrument, other reference materials dealing with facial morphology are available for more in-depth information, and readers are referred to these publications (Jung, 1989; Shprintzen, 1997; Shprintzen, 2000; Shprintzen & Witzel, 1993).

Examining the Structures of the Oral Mechanism

Lips

The lips are the most visible of the articulators used in producing speech and are important in the ingestion of food (Perlman & Christensen, 1997). Lip articulation is a component in the production of a number of vowel and consonant speech sounds (MacKay, 1978). For example, the lips are the primary constriction in the formation of the bilabial plosives /p/ and /b/ and nasal /m/, and the lower lip and upper teeth serve as the point of articulation for the fricative cognates /f/ and /v/. In addition to speech production, the lips in conjunction with the tongue are important structures in the oral preparation of a food bolus and oral transport of the bolus through the oral cavity in preparation for triggering the pharyngeal swallow (Perlman & Christensen, 1997).

The lips are composed of muscle and glandular tissue. The outside or exterior skin surface of the lips terminates into an elevated white line known as the mucocutaneous ridge. The landmark curve of the upper lip is known as *Cupid's bow* (Brescia, 1971). The red zone between the outer skin portion of the lip and mucous membrane is the vermilion zone. The orbicularis oris muscle is the major muscle of lip function. It is an unpaired muscle that forms a complete circle around the oral opening. Cranial nerve (CN) VII provides motor innervation, whereas sensory feedback is provided by afferent fibers of CN V. (Appendix 6B provides a summary of CN function for the oral musculature.)

Mason (1994) describes the typical resting relationship of the lips as meeting together with an open space between the upper and lower front teeth. Generally, the lower lip covers approximately 2–3 mm of the upper incisors. The open distance between the posterior teeth in the rest position is also approximately 2–3 mm. This space is referred to as *freeway space*.

There can be a wide range in acceptable muscle function of the lips because precise articulations are not necessary (Spriestersbach et al., 1978). Asymmetric appearance, such as in the case of a cleft lip repair, is not a direct indicator of a lip mobility problem. Spriestersbach et al. (1961) suggest that lip scarring and the resultant deviations usually are not a major factor in the speech problems of persons with cleft lip and palate. Shprintzen and Witzel (1993) recommend that the practitioner study the upper and lower lips, because anomalies of the lips are very common and can be a feature of many different birth syndromes.

An upper lip that on visual inspection appears "tight" and is immobile may be the result of a restricted labial frenum. A tongue blade or gloved finger may be used to view the labial frenum and determine if its attachment with the alveolus and the inside portion of the upper lip is restricted. In some cases, the client may need to be seen by an oral surgeon for treatment if a restriction is noted.

Some clients have difficulty closing the lips because of maxillary or mandibular dental or skeletal problems and exhibit a chronic lips-apart resting posture. Clients who experience difficulty closing the lips with observable strain of the mentalis muscle have "lip incompetence" (Mason, 1994). In other cases, the lips-apart resting posture is not a sign of lip incompetence but may be a behavioral manifestation of an earlier problem with the nasal airway obstruction (Kellum, 1994). A number of investigators have speculated that the lips-apart posture is the result of a restricted nasal airway during early childhood. In some cases, the problem has resolved, but the lips-apart resting posture is maintained because of habit and hypotonic labial muscle tissue. Practitioners should be mindful of the fact that lip incompetence is often present in children to approximately 13 years of age because the lips have not completely developed. Mason (1994) indicates that the lips continue to develop in the vertical dimension until approximately 17 years of age; however, lip competence in most clients is achieved by age 12–13 years.

Other problems with lip posture and movement may be the result of damage to the nervous system. The neurologic disorders of apraxia and dysarthria are collectively known as *motor speech disorders* (Darley, 1978; Duffy, 1995). The client with apraxia of speech exhibits difficulty in sequencing and executing articulatory movements. There is difficulty in programming the movement patterns requisite for the execution of the muscles in the volitional act of speaking (Duffy, 1995). Conversely, the dysarthric client has a motor speech disorder that may manifest in problems such as muscular weakness, lack of muscle tone, uncoordinated movement, reduced speed of movement, or some combination (Darley et al., 1975). Darley et al. (1975) identify definitive speech symptoms that correspond to different types of neural damage at the central or peripheral nervous system levels. A client with bilateral lip involvement of a lower motor neuron type frequently presents with a particular posture at rest. Often in such cases, there is a broad weakness of the facial muscles. The labial opening is displaced downward proximate to the mandibular teeth along with a downward curving of the upper and lower lips. In addition, the nasolabial fold is accentuated (Bosma, 1976). This type of problem can be very serious for speech and feeding skills because lip function is deficient.

Generally, there is an observable asymmetry of the lip at rest in the case of unilateral lower motor neuron involvement. The affected side is lower than the unaffected side of the lip (Darley et al., 1975). During movement activities, the unaffected side moves upward and laterally, but a unilateral lesion typically has little effect on the production of labial articulations.

One needs to keep in mind that this narrative summarizes some of the diagnostic markers of dysarthria. Differential diagnosis is established through careful scrutiny with a battery of evaluative instruments to isolate the specific disorder type (Duffy, 1995). This warning is also appropriate for clients whose symptoms appear to be consistent with apraxia of speech. The characteristic features of apraxia of speech in adults are articulatory inaccuracy and, to a lesser degree, prosodic speech differences (Darley, 1978). Some clients also have problems carrying out isolated voluntary nonspeech movements or sequences of movements (LaPointe & Wertz, 1974), and such information can be useful in diagnosis. Interested readers are referred to excellent texts (Caruso & Strand, 1999; Darley et al., 1975; Duffy, 1995; Love, 1992; Yorkston et al., 1999) for in-depth information on motor speech disorders.

A final problem that may be noted during labial assessment is a problem with saliva control or drooling. There are two different consistencies of saliva that are produced by the salivary glands (Johnson & Scott, 1993). Serous or watery saliva is secreted mainly by the parotid glands, whereas the sublingual and submandibular glands secrete mucoid saliva. Perlman et al. (1997) indicate that drooling is a frequent problem encountered in younger clients with developmental disorders such as cerebral palsy and older clients with acquired neurologic deficits. Impaired oral sensation and weakness of the orbicularis oris muscle are often causative factors of drooling.

Tongue

The tongue is the most important oral structure of speech and swallowing. It functions as the major articulator for many speech sounds (Daniloff, 1973; Perkins & Kent, 1986). Tongue movements modify the configuration of the oral cavity, thus changing the resonating features of the vocal tract. Tongue articulations can completely occlude the vocal tract, partially constrict it, or assume other shapes that can alter the breath stream during speech production. Kier and Smith (1985) indicate that the tongue is a muscular hydrostat lacking primary skeletal support. Intrinsic and extrinsic muscles play the major role in support and movement of the tongue. The major feature of a muscular hydrostat is that it is capable of assuming different shapes without changing its volume. Suffice it to say that the tongue is a highly mobile articulator that is capable of making very fine muscular adjustments.

The tongue is also a key structure in the feeding process. It functions in both the oral preparation and oral transport of a food bolus (Perlman & Christensen, 1997). Logemann (1998) indicates that movement of the bolus during oral preparation varies as a function of food viscosity and the degree of oral manipulation used in tasting a particular food. Individuals use different strategies to manipulate the bolus, but in each case, the tongue is an important structure in terms of both movement and sensory feedback.

Anatomically, the tongue is divided into the tip, blade, dorsum, and root or tongue base (Daniloff, 1973). According to Mason (1994), the growth of the tongue corresponds to the neural growth curve. Generally, most tongue growth takes place by 8 years of age, and very little growth is expected after 12 years of age.

The tongue is located in the floor of the mouth and is attached to a number of adjacent structures (Kaplin, 1971). The inferior surface is attached to the mandible, and the lingual frenum elevates to connect in midline with the underside of the tongue. The upper surface of the tongue is separated into lateral aspects by the longitudinal median sulcus. The sulcus extends posteriorly to a pitlike structure that is the foramen cecum. Laterally and forward to the foramen cecum is a groovelike landmark known as the *sulcus terminalis*.

There are eight muscles of the tongue that are divided into intrinsic and extrinsic muscle groups; however, it is difficult to trace the course of the various muscles because they are so interwoven within the tongue. The various muscles, categorized by group, are included in Table 6.1.

TABLE 6.1   Intrinsic and extrinsic lingual muscles

Intrinsic muscles of the tongue (paired muscles)
    Superior longitudinal
    Inferior longitudinal
    Transverse
    Vertical
Extrinsic muscles of the tongue
    Genioglossus
    Styloglossus
    Palatoglossus
    Hyoglossus

The intrinsic muscles of the tongue are paired muscles, and they act to move and shape the tongue for various speech and nonspeech functions (Daniloff, 1973). Zemlin (1998) indicates that contraction of the superior longitudinal muscles shortens the tongue or acts to curl the edges and tip upward. The inferior longitudinal muscles also shorten the tongue and depress the tip of the tongue downward. Narrowing and elongation of the tongue are achieved through contractions of the transverse muscles, whereas the vertical muscles function to flatten the tongue.

The extrinsic muscles of the tongue originate from other structures and insert into the body of the tongue (Zemlin, 1998). The genioglossus is a very large muscle that accounts for a significant part of the bulk of the tongue. Contractions of muscle fibers allow the tongue to assume a number of different positions. The posterior fibers pull the tongue forward to achieve protrusion of the tip outside the mouth. Tongue backing is accomplished through action of the anterior fibers; contraction of all genioglossus muscle fibers draws the tongue downward. Activity of the styloglossus muscles moves the tongue upward and backward. It is thought that contraction of the styloglossus muscles may also help in pulling the lateral margins of the tongue upward.

The glossopalatine is included with the extrinsic tongue muscles, but it is also classified as a *muscle of the palate* in some texts. In the latter case, it is classified as the *palatoglossus muscle*. Activity of the glossopalatine muscle is believed to be responsible for elevation of the back of the tongue. Moon and Kuehn (1996) present a comprehensive review of oral anatomy and physiology and indicate that the glossopalatine muscles participate in tongue elevation and lowering of the velum; however, the actions of the muscles are dependent on whether the tongue or velum is more fixed at the time of contraction. Contractions of the hyoglossus muscles pull the tongue in a backward and downward position. It is also thought that the hyoglossus muscles assist in hyoid bone elevation.

Efferent innervation to all intrinsic lingual muscles and to a majority of the extrinsic and infrahyoid muscles is provided by the hypoglossal nerve (CN 12) (Perkins & Kent, 1986). Branches of the trigeminal (CN V), facial (CN VII), and glossopharyngeal (CN IX) nerves convey afferent information, such as sensation and taste.

Observation of the tongue at rest is conducted with the patient's mouth open and tongue remaining within the oral cavity. Darley et al. (1975) suggest that the examiner inspect the tongue to ascertain if it is normal in appearance and shape. Characteristic clinical indicators that may be indicative of neurologic involvement include furrowing along the tongue surface or a tongue that looks reduced in size. When there is unilateral involvement, the affected side may appear smaller or furrowed in shape. Duffy (1995) states that muscles deprived of their neurologic input gradually atrophy. During the beginning stages of muscle atrophy, motor units innervating the muscle fibers may fire spontaneously and present as slight movements or twitches on the surface of the skin. The observable muscular activity is known as a *fasciculation*.

Although it is rare, the examiner may see clients with aglossia, or the absence of a tongue. The disorder is typically caused by some congenital or acquired problem (Ewanowski & Saxman, 1980). Medical treatment for oral cancers or acquired injuries often requires the excision of a portion of lingual tissue or a total glossectomy. The magnitude of the disease process determines whether a partial or total glossectomy is needed. The client's competence in using the tongue for speech and nonspeech functions depends on the compensatory skills that he or she may develop.

Relative judgments of tongue size are problematic for the examiner, because the tongue is situated in the oral cavity space and bounded by the maxilla and mandible. A tongue that seems unusually large may actually be normal in mass if the mandible or lower jaw is limited in size. *Microglossia* is a term used to describe an abnormally small tongue, whereas *macroglossia* is used to describe an unusually large tongue. When the lower jaw is smaller than expected, the tongue may be in a more posterior position. Such tongue posture can hinder nasal breathing, a condition known as *glossoptosis*. Shprintzen and Witzel (1993) indicate that malformations of the tongue occur less frequently than anomalies of the palate; however, there are syndromes that include characteristics such as tongue anomalies. For example, macroglossia is often associated with Beckwith-Wiedemann syndrome, and microglossia is frequently found in individuals with hypoglossia-hypodactyly sequence. Clefting of the tongue or lobulation is a condition found infrequently, but is found in a number of syndromes like oral–facial–digital syndrome, type I. Further information concerning birth malformations from the perspective of the speech-language pathologist is available in a number of excellent texts (Jung, 1989; Shprintzen, 1997; Shprintzen, 2000).

The lingual frenum is studied by instructing the patient to elevate the tongue when the mouth is open. There is no particular method for evaluating the potential effects of the lingual frenum on tongue mobility. However, it should be noted that descriptions of a restricted lingual frenum have been found in association with disorders of speech and vegetative function, such as eating. The differential diagnosis of ankyloglossia or tongue tie is a problematic task for the practitioner. Symptoms may include difficulty making tongue tip contact with the alveolar ridge, and the tongue tip or the anterior lateral surface of the tongue may assume a heart-shaped appearance on protrusion between the central incisors

(Spriestersbach et al., 1978). Some investigators provide guidelines for assessment. For example, Peterson-Falzone (1982) feels that a restricted lingual frenum is not problematic for a client who can raise the tongue tip to the alveolar ridge with the mouth one-fourth to one-third open and sweep the outer surface of the lips to remove bits of food. Warden (1991) also recommends that the diagnosis of ankyloglossia be based on observing certain movement positions of the tongue. If a client can protrude the tongue more than 1–2 mm past the mandibular incisors or touch the hard palate with the tongue tip, the lingual frenum is not judged to be restrictive. According to Warden, a diagnosis cannot be rendered until such time as the child has acquired his or her primary dentition. This is due to the fact that the tongue tip is not fully developed in the infant and appears short on visual observation.

Fletcher and Meldrum (1968) developed a measurement technique for quantifying lingual dimensions, but there is no normative database that would permit comparison among clients. Williams and Waldron (1985) systematically studied lingual function and collected client data on speech tasks and various lingual dimensions using procedures reported by Fletcher and Meldrum. The examiners were unable to develop guidelines for diagnosing ankyloglossia, but it is clear from their report that a restricted lingual frenum requiring intervention such as surgery is a rare occurrence.

Overall tongue mobility can be studied by having the client carry out movement tasks. A unilateral neurologic involvement presents with deviation of the tongue to the impaired side (Darley et al., 1975); however, the significance of the impairment on articulation is generally not great. A client with bilateral involvement, on the other hand, demonstrates overall movement difficulties and articulatory impairment. Duffy (1995) indicates that there is a general imprecision of consonant articulation and distorted vowel sound productions. A client who has apraxia of speech may also have an oral apraxia and have problems in executing nonspeech lingual movements.

Examiners should also identify any oral myofunctional variables that may be observed during the examination. Kellum (1994) cautions practitioners that a broad perspective must be adopted in evaluating a client with potential oral myofunctional disorders (OMD). The practitioner must study oral rest postures, habit patterns, and swallowing patterns of the client. Some lingual OMD variables of diagnostic significance are linguadental rest and lingual swallow postures; lingual movement before and after the swallow; lingual movement during speech and nonspeech tasks, such as reduced tongue-tip elevation and retroflexion; and general incoordination of lingual movement.

Mason (1994) indicates that the tongue can influence other oral structures, such as the teeth. A habitual front tongue carriage can obstruct eruption of the front teeth for children who are in the mixed stage of dental development. Furthermore, the anterior posturing of the tongue combined with a mandible-open position beyond expected freeway space may cause posterior teeth to erupt early and ultimately lead to difficulties with dental occlusion. If the resting posture of the tongue is habitually forward, with the posterior and lateral margins of the tongue extended over the lower back teeth, the upper teeth continue to erupt, but the lower teeth are hindered from erupting totally. Current thinking is that the movement of tongue thrust may aggravate an existing malocclusion, but the tongue thrust is probably not the cause of the malocclusion.

Hale and her colleagues (1992) examined a number of OMD variables in a group of 133 second-graders. The OMD study variables include

1. Lips-apart and open-mouth resting position, as examined during a listening activity
2. Accuracy of production and articulatory position of the lingua-alveolar consonant speech sounds
3. Tongue posture at rest when required to face the examiner and relax
4. Tongue swallow patterns during the ingestion of water

The results suggest that rest and swallow postures may affect or are affected by oral motor behavior such as diadochokinetic rates—that is, the authors felt that there was a relationship between speech and non-speech oral behaviors, but they were not clear as to the agent responsible for the influence. The practitioner must be alert to these conditions and is directed to current literature pertaining to issues of OMD for further information (ASHA, 1991a; ASHA, 1993; Ferketic & Gardner, 1994).

The tongue is also an important component in deglutition. Lingual management of a bolus is necessary in the oral preparatory and oral phase of swallowing (Logemann, 1983). During oral preparation, there is a rotary, lateral motion of the tongue and mandible for a bolus consistency that requires chewing. The teeth and tongue act to move the bolus within the oral cavity and mix it with saliva. After chewing has been completed, the tongue forms a bolus, holds it in position for a brief period of time, and begins to move it posteriorly. The midline of the tongue presses the bolus against the hard palate in a sequential manner as it is moved to the back of the mouth in preparation of triggering the pharyngeal swallow.

Teeth

The teeth are the main stationary articulators of the oral speech mechanism. The teeth function as a place of primary articulation for several English phonemes, such as the /f/ and /v/ and /ø/ and /ð/ cognates. The teeth, especially the anterior incisors, serve as fixed structures against which air turbulence is created to produce high-frequency acoustic energy, as evidenced in the production of lingual fricative speech sounds. Moreover, the molars serve to confine lateral and posterior tongue placement for sounds such as the liquids /l/, /r/, and the plosive pair /k, g/. Zemlin (1998) states that the teeth play an integral part in the production of all English phonemes, including vowels.

The human dental arch consists of primary or deciduous teeth and permanent teeth. Depending on the age of the individual, the arch may consist of primary teeth, permanent teeth, or be mixed in composition. The deciduous and permanent dental arches develop during the embryonic growth of the human fetus, but the deciduous teeth erupt initially and are gradually supplanted by the permanent teeth. There is a great deal of variability across individuals regarding the age of eruption of specific teeth; however, there is usually an anterior-to-posterior eruption of teeth. First, the anterior teeth (incisors) erupt, followed by the cuspids (canines) and then molars. The only major difference to this tendency is that the first permanent molars tend to be the initial permanent teeth to erupt. Generally, the deciduous or baby teeth erupt between the ages of 7.5 months to 2 years of age (Sicher & DuBrul, 1975). The teeth of the permanent dental arch begin to erupt at age 6 and end at approximately 21 years of age, but if the third molars ("wisdom teeth") are not included, the typical range of permanent teeth eruption is between 6 and 13 years of age. Table 6.2 lists the deciduous and permanent dental arches.

The location of individual teeth can be categorized in relation to approximate soft structures. The lips (*labial aspect*), cheeks (*buccal aspect*) on the outside of the teeth, and tongue (*lingual aspect*) on the inside of the teeth are terms used to indicate placement. With the anterior center of the dental arch as the median reference point, each tooth can also be located with respect to location or movement either toward (mesial) or away from (distal) the median reference.

In addition to observing and reporting locations of individual teeth within the upper (maxillary) and lower (mandibular) dental arches, the dentition is also examined in reference to the bite relationship between the upper and lower dental arches. The association of the biting surfaces of the teeth in the closed position is occlusion.

The deciduous or primary dental arch contains central incisors, lateral incisors, cuspids (canines), first molars, and second molars. There are a total of 20 teeth: 10 located in the maxillary arch and 10 in the mandibular arch. It is to be noted that the maxillary arch is somewhat larger than the mandibular arch and typically overlaps on the anterior and lateral sides in normal occlusion.

The occlusion of the upper and lower first molars is used to examine posterior occlusion. In the expected relationship of the permanent dental arches, the mandibular first molar is slightly anterior or one-half cusp ahead of the maxillary first molar. Practitioners are cautioned that in the deciduous and mixed dentition arches, the first molars frequently present in an end-to-end relation. Examiners need to keep in mind that children between the ages of 6 to 13 are usually in the mixed dentition stage. There are 16 teeth in each of the permanent dental arches. Each arch consists of the central incisors, lat-

TABLE 6.2   Teeth of the deciduous and permanent dental arches from anterior to posterior position

Deciduous teeth	Permanent teeth
Central incisor	Central incisor
Lateral incisor	Lateral incisor
Cuspid	Cuspid
First molar	First bicuspid
Second molar	Second bicuspid
—	First molar
—	Second molar
—	Third molar (wisdom)

eral incisors, cuspids (canines), first bicuspids (premolars), second bicuspids (premolars), first molars, second molars, and third molars.

Deviations of the dental arches are described as *malocclusions*. Malocclusions are differences in the bite relationships between the maxillary and mandibular dental arches. Most speech-language pathologists are familiar with Angle's (1907) three classes of malocclusion that use the first molars as the reference point. Angle's class I malocclusion (neutroclusion) is a normal first molar bite relationship with occlusal problems of the anterior teeth. Class II malocclusion (distoclusion) is the most frequent malocclusion observed in the general population. The maxilla or upper jaw is protruded anteriorly to the mandible. Class II malocclusions are classified into two types. In class II, division 1, the maxillary incisors project outwardly (labioverted); however, a class II, division 2 malocclusion consists of retruded (linguaverted) maxillary central incisors with labially and mesially tipped lateral incisors. Class III malocclusion (mesioocclusion) is a condition wherein the maxilla is retruded or retracted in relation to the mandible. Malocclusions may result from dental or skeletal-based problems. Practitioners should be careful to refer to a dental specialist so that the causal basis for the occlusal problem may be identified and treated.

Occlusal problems of the anterior teeth occur quite often and may be noted with or without molar malocclusions. If the maxillary incisors cover more than one-third of the mandibular incisors, the condition is known as *close bite*. The converse—in which the biting edges of the incisors do not overlap (as viewed from the front) when the molars are in occlusion—is an *open bite*. An open bite may present bilaterally or unilaterally, depending on the extent of the anterior malocclusion (Zemlin, 1998). When the maxillary incisors extend anteriorly beyond the mandibular incisors, an *overbite* is present. Some practitioners also describe the condition as an *overjet*. If a tooth in the upper dental arch is oriented to the interior lingual surface of a lower tooth, or a segment of the upper and lower dental arches are situated in such a position, a *crossbite* is present (Mason, 1994).

The importance of malocclusions in explaining defective speech production is ambiguous; consequently, it is difficult to establish causal relationships between dental structure and speech function (Mason, 1994; Peterson-Falzone, 1982). In a comprehensive review of the literature, Winitz (1969) expresses the opinion that occlusal deviations are not clearly related to articulatory production errors. However, there are some data that furnish support for a relationship between occlusal problems and articulation errors. Ruscello et al. (1985) summarize a number of representative investigations that examine speech production before and after orthognathic surgery. The patients had different malocclusions, and 72% of the clients had articulatory production errors before surgical intervention. The most frequent errors were described as distortions and were indicative of phonetically based problems. The sibilant sound class and the /s/ speech sound in particular were most often identified as defective across studies. After surgery, approximately 82% of the patients with preoperative errors reduced or eliminated completely their articulation errors. Readers should be mindful that in most cases, the reported errors were typically mild in severity and did not significantly hinder intelligibility. Bloomer (1971) feels that distocclusion is most frequently associated with articulation errors. Nevertheless, the sounds most frequently reported to be in error, regardless of the type of malocclusion, are the sibilants /s/, /z/, /ʃ/, /tʃ/, and /dʒ/, and occasionally the speech sounds /f/, /v/, /ø/, and /ð/ (Bloomer, 1971; Luchsinger & Arnold, 1965; Winitz, 1969).

The relationship between articulatory production errors and malocclusion of the anterior teeth is similarly problematic, but there are some conditional findings that emerge from reviews. Bloomer (1971), Peterson-Falzone (1982), Starr (1971), and Winitz (1969) all indicate that open-bite malocclusions are more likely to coexist with /s/ and /z/ articulation errors than by chance occurrence.

There are some additional factors that also need to be kept in mind before the significance of any occlusal problem is established. For example, Mason and Proffit (1974) cite a U.S. Public Health Service study that identifies open bite as occurring approximately five times more frequently among African American than white school children. Orthodontists frequently identify anterior occlusal problems, such as incisor protrusion and open bite, as symptoms of tongue thrusting. During dental treatment, orthodontists frequently obtain the assistance of speech-language pathologists for the purpose of retraining swallowing patterns and minimizing unnecessary lingual pressure against the teeth. The rationale for oral motor intervention is to retain correct incisor location after orthodontia is finished. Many cases exhibit a ø/s (frontal lisp) misarticulation, and the articulatory component is presumed to be a speech sequela of tongue thrusting. As mentioned previously, the current position is that the functional movement of tongue thrust may exacerbate a malocclusion, but the tongue thrust is likely not the causal agent of the malocclusion.

Generally, the misalignment of single teeth does not have a significant effect on speech production. Extensive reviews of the clinical and research literature by various investigators (Bloomer, 1971; Luchsinger & Arnold, 1965; Starr, 1971; Winitz, 1969) imply that subjects with dental irregularities as a group tend to have more frequent misarticulations than individuals without dental problems. Once again, /s/ and other sibilant distortions are the most commonly identified production errors.

The relationship of missing teeth to articulation remains equivocal. Bloomer (1971) writes that loss of all the teeth may result in fricative distortion. Another issue of considerable controversy is the potential effect of dental spacing by expected shedding of central incisors on speech production errors. Snow (1961) reports that missing or maligned central incisors negatively influence the production characteristics of fricative sounds, principally /s/ and /z/. Bankson and Byrne (1962) found that missing front teeth had a negative impact on /s/ but not /z/, /f/, and /ʃ/ in kindergarten and first-grade children. In most cases, the normal shedding of the incisors has no long-term effect on speech production skills, but /s/ production may be affected temporarily.

It can also be concluded that without other intervening variables, dental anomalies rarely have a serious impact on articulation (Starr, 1971). Nevertheless, Peterson-Falzone (1982) also examined the issue of dental problems and concluded that the practitioner must examine speech production skills very carefully to establish which errors are developmental and which may be related to any existing dental condition. Dental problems require referral to a dental specialist for examination and possible treatment (Trost-Cardamone, 1995). Terms for describing various dental conditions have been compiled and listed in Table 6.3.

Finally, there are clients who may have artificial teeth, dental bridges, complete dentures, or various prosthetic devices that are part of the dental arch or are attached to the dental arch. The practitioner should describe the dental appliance and question the client to determine if it has some adverse effect on oral function.

Hard Palate

The hard palate or bony roof of the mouth is a structure that is very important in speech production and deglutition (Daniloff, 1973; Logemann, 1998). Tongue and hard palate articulations can occlude the vocal tract completely, or partial constrictions can create an orifice of restricted dimension. For example, production of the fricative sound /ʃ/ entails the creation of a narrow constriction of the vocal tract with the tongue and palate. The tip of the tongue is raised in the area of the palate that is just behind the alveolar ridge. Air is then forced through the small constriction with a high-frequency, noisy fricative sound being produced. The hard palate also serves as a partial separation of the oral cavity and nasal cavity.

The outer surface of the hard palate is composed of mucous membrane (Zemlin, 1998). The membrane is very pronounced on the posterior edge of the alveolar area, appearing as a ridgelike configuration. The ridges (or rugae) typically decrease in prominence with age. A midline raphe or suture is present when viewing the hard palate. The midline raphe starts just behind the rugae and courses the entire length of the hard palate. In some individuals, particularly of Northern European extraction, a pronounced longitudinal ridge or bump (the palatine torus) is seen along the margins of the midline raphe (Cassell & Elkadi, 1995).

The bony composition of the hard palate consists of the palatine processes of the maxilla and the horizontal plates of the palatine bones. Zemlin (1998) indicates that the palatine processes form approximately 75% of the bony hard palate, and the palatine bone plates compose the posterior 25% of the palate. The palatine bone plates come together in midline to

TABLE 6.3   Terms for describing various dental conditions

Anodontia: Failure of tooth or teeth to form; congenital absence of teeth

Bruxism: Teeth grinding or clenching

Diastema: Wide spaces between teeth

Ectopic tooth: A tooth that is misplaced

Microdontia: A tooth (or teeth) that is small in size

Missing teeth: Spaces where individual teeth should be present

Oligodontia: Fewer than the normal complement of teeth

Supernumerary tooth: An additional tooth

form the posterior nasal spine. The soft palate or muscular portion of the roof of the mouth is affixed to the posterior margins of the palatine bones. Sensory innervation of the hard palate is furnished by the trigeminal nerve (CN V).

The contour of the palate is one of an arched or dome-shaped structure in transverse and anterior/posterior orientations. Of particular import to the speech-language pathologist is the transverse arch configuration. The height and width of the palatal vault should be studied for relative appearance. Spriestersbach et al. (1978) indicate that the palatal configuration of most individuals is usually adequate for communication purposes. However, Keuhn (1982) cautions that anomalous palatal arch configurations may negatively influence the resonance characteristics of the vocal tract. This is very plausible, especially for those clients who present with craniofacial malformations or acquired injuries associated with oral cancer or injuries.

Witzel (1995) describes some different palatal arch configurations and discusses potential speech and resonance sequelae. She suggests that aberrant hard palate configurations may cause tongue position and tongue posture changes and adversely influence the generation of airflow through the oral cavity. A client with a very low, flat-shaped palate may have difficulty with tongue-palate contacts and oral resonance. Further, clients with a high palate and narrow arch configuration may encounter problems with lingua-palatal articulation and may report food sticking in the palatal arch. Interested readers may consult a number of excellent reviews that contain information regarding malformations of the hard palate and possible consequences on speech, resonance, and other oral physiology (Carey et al., 1992; Peterson-Falzone, 1987).

Examination of the hard palate may also disclose differences such as open clefts, scar tissue, fistulae, or other malformations. Practitioners may examine young infants before surgical repair of a cleft palate. In some cases, surgical closure of a cleft palate is performed in stages; consequently, a portion of the cleft remains unrepaired for a period of time, and the defect is temporarily obturated (McWilliams et al., 1990; Seagle, 1997).

Persons who have undergone palatal repair may exhibit visible scarring that is the result of corrective surgery. A palatal fistula may be present in clients who have had surgical correction of the hard palate. Fistulae are tissue breakdowns resulting from partial wound dehiscence at the site of surgical repair. Ewanowski and Saxman (1980) recommend that practitioners also examine the space between the upper lip and alveolar ridge because nasolabial fistulae may be present in some cases. Fistula can cause oronasal coupling with client symptoms such as hypernasality, nasal air emission, and feeding problems, or the fistula may be asymptomatic. If a fistula is problematic as determined through assessment, surgery or obturation may be used to correct the defect. Oral cancer patients may present with substantial palatal defects as a result of surgery and require palatal obturators.

Although primarily conceptualized as a defect of the soft palate, a submucous cleft palate can also affect the hard palate. The stigmata of a submucous cleft are generally listed as bifid uvula, midline muscle defect of the palatal muscles, and a posterior nasal spine deformity (Bradley, 1997). Bardach and Salyer (1995) state that the cleft may encompass a portion or the entire soft palate, including the posterior part of the hard palate. If the submucous cleft includes the hard palate, it is a bony defect of the posterior nasal spine. Mason and Simon (1977) indicate that the posterior nasal spine defect is present in most cases of submucous cleft. Examination of the posterior nasal spine for the bony anomaly can be carried out by finger palpation. It should be noted that a submucous cleft may be identified, but medical or prosthetic intervention is not necessary in cases wherein the defect is not symptomatic for speech or feeding problems. If a submucous cleft is identified with accompanying speech or nonspeech symptoms, the appropriate referral for further assessment would need to be made to establish a treatment plan.

Soft Palate

The soft palate or velum is a muscular valve that functions to separate the oral cavity from the nasal cavity during both speech and nonspeech activities (Ruscello, 1997). Its muscular movements are conducted in connection with the lateral and posterior pharyngeal walls. Moon and Kuehn (1996) studied the coordinated movement of the velopharyngeal complex and identified two basic patterns of movement. One is soft palate elevation to the posterior pharyngeal wall and then lowering away from the posterior pharyngeal wall. The second is the mesial movement of the lateral pharyngeal walls. Taken together, the contributions of the muscles create the sphincteric action of the velopharyngeal valve. Some speakers may also use additional movement patterns—such as anterior movement of the posterior pharyngeal wall and bulging of the nasal surface of the velum—during speech production. The velopharyngeal valve functions to block the nasal cavity during the production of oral speech sounds and allows nasal coupling during the articulation of nasal sounds. The velar on/off portrayal is somewhat of an oversimplification, because there are variations in velopharyngeal closure as a result of coarticulatory influences that occur in continuous speech (Hixon & Abbs, 1980).

The velum (or soft palate) and the lateral and posterior pharyngeal wall muscles are the muscle groups that constitute the velopharyngeal mechanism (Moon & Kuehn, 1997). The velum attaches anteriorly to the palatine bones of the hard palate (Zemlin, 1998). Muscle fibers on the lateral aspects of the soft palate mix with fibers of the superior constrictor muscle, one of the three constrictor muscles of the pharynx. The paired muscles of the soft palate are the levator veli palatini, tensor veli palatini, musculus uvulae, palatoglossus, palatopharyngeus, superior pharyngeal constrictor, and salpingopharyngeus. Electromyography studies of the velopharyngeal network have been completed, and data suggest that the levator veli palatini is the major palatal muscle in velar elevation (Fritzell, 1969), and differences in velar height may be a function of variations in the degree of levator muscle action. Data reported by Moon and Keuhn (1997) indicate that the levator functions in combination with the palatoglossus and palatopharyngeus muscles. The interplay among the muscles strongly suggests that velar elevation is a complex muscular activity. Similarly, lowering of the velum is conceptualized as a complex muscular activity; however, the muscular components have not been totally delineated. Current research suggests that the palatoglossus has a role in the lowering of the velum, and muscular actions of the palatopharyngeus, along with suppression of the levator muscles, have also been identified in electromyographic studies.

Mesial movement of the lateral pharyngeal walls is one of the muscular forces that frequently acts in velopharyngeal closure during speech, but the mechanism accountable for lateral wall movement has not been identified. Contemporary explanations of velopharyngeal closure imply that mesial activity of the lateral pharyngeal walls may be due to activity of the levator muscles or the superior constrictor muscle. Contributions of the posterior pharyngeal wall in closure activity differ markedly among speakers. Some exhibit minimal displacement of the posterior pharyngeal wall, whereas others demonstrate extensive excursion from rest. In some individuals, there is a marked displacement or bulging out of the muscle. This is referred to as *Passavant's ridge*, and it has been reported in both normal speakers and those with cleft palate. Some researchers feel that the superior constrictor muscle is the agent responsible for the bulging movement; however, others feel that the horizontal fibers of the palatopharyngeus muscles are responsible for the bulging of the posterior pharyngeal wall (Moon and Kuehn, 1997).

The glossopharyngeal (CN IX) and vagus (CN X) nerves provide motor innervation to the velopharyngeal mechanism. Cassell and Elkadi (1995) indicate that the facial (CN VII) and hypoglossal (CN XII) nerves may also contribute to the motor innervation of the velopharynx. Sensory or afferent feedback is provided by branches of the trigeminal (CN V) nerve.

If the client has had a secondary surgical repair of the palate, there may be differences in palatal anatomy on inspection. Shprintzen (1995) furnishes an excellent description of secondary surgical procedures that have been designed to improve velopharyngeal closure for speech. One of the most frequent is the pharyngeal flap, and there are a number of variations of the surgical procedure that have been reported in the literature. A tissue flap is placed surgically inferiorly or superiorly in relation to the soft palate. An inferior-based pharyngeal flap can generally be examined visually, because the flap of tissue is dissected from the posterior pharyngeal wall below the level of the soft palate. A superior-based flap cannot be examined visually, because it is sutured to the nasal side of the soft palate above the plane of intraoral view.

A submucous cleft of the soft palate may be observed when conducting a visual inspection of the soft palate. The defect may include a bifid uvula, a muscular deficiency of the soft palate, and a bony defect of the posterior nasal spine. Submucous clefts of the soft palate are often difficult to diagnose but may be exposed after the client has undergone an adenoidectomy (Spriestersbach et al., 1978). Data reported by Mason and Simon (1977) suggest the presence of a bifid uvula in approximately one of 75 individuals who are assessed. As mentioned previously, a submucous cleft may or may not be symptomatic for speech or feeding problems (Ewanoski & Saxman, 1980).

If the possibility of a neurologic impairment exists, the soft palate may appear asymmetric (Wilson-Pauwels et al., 1988). Aronson (1980) states that some clients may exhibit asymmetries as a result of tonsillectomy removal and consequent scarring; however, most asymmetries observed are indicators of neurologic disease. When movement of the soft palate is noted during speech production, excursion is noted to estimate velopharyngeal closure for speech. Asymmetry of palatal activity suggests the possibility of unilateral neurologic involvement. On observation, the affected side remains lower than the unaffected side. In the case of bilateral involvement, there may be limited excursion to closure or a total lack of movement. For example, in cases of bilateral neurologic involvement of the lower motor neuron, the soft palate remains lowered, lacks expected arching, and is proximate to the tongue dorsum (Darley et al., 1975).

Velopharyngeal incompetence can severely affect speech. Vocal quality may be hypernasal, because there is coupling between the oral and nasal cavities. Moreover, the production of oral pressure sounds (plosives, fricatives, and affricates) may be produced with coexisting audible nasal emission, or the client may develop posterior articulations, such as glottal stops. There may also be feeding issues, because of nasal reflux during the ingestion of certain food viscosities like liquids.

There are several screening tests that have been developed to examine velopharyngeal closure. For example, the nasal flutter or nasal pinch test is a screening measure that helps in establishing if additional instrumental testing and referral are necessary. The client is instructed to sustain production of the vowel /u/ while alternately opening and closing the nares. A client with appropriate closure does not demonstrate voice quality changes under the two different conditions. A client with a closure deficit is typically hypernasal with the nostrils open and then exhibits a voice quality change with the nostrils occluded. In some cases, the quality change is not perceived, but nasal vibration can be felt with the fingers.

The modified tongue-anchor technique is another tool that has been used for screening purposes (Fox & Johns, 1970). The patient is instructed to "puff up the cheeks" with air while the tongue is protruded and the nares are occluded with digital pressure. The examiner releases the nares and notes if the patient can keep the cheeks inflated. Velopharyngeal closure is assumed if the patient can maintain the cheeks-inflated condition, whereas lack of closure would be associated with the inability of the patient to maintain the inflated condition.

Oral cancer patients may wear appliances to obturate a palatal defect and assist with speech and feeding skills. Other clients may be fitted with prosthetic appliances because of such problems as cleft palate or neurologic disease. The two appliances used most often are speech bulbs and palatal lifts (Rosen & Bzoch, 1997). Leeper et al. (1993) provide a cogent discussion of the construction of prosthetic speech appliances and their role in improving speech production and other oral functions. A prosthetic appliance typically is made up of a palatal base plate that is molded to fit the oral anatomy and attach to the dentition. If there is a defect of the hard palate, such as a fistula, the appliance closes the defect. Expansion of the palatal plate or base is done to aid in the achievement of velopharyngeal closure for speech. A pharyngeal section is added to function as a speech bulb or palatal lift. A speech bulb furnishes partial obturation of the velopharyngeal area so that in interaction with the muscles of the velopharyngeal complex, closure of the mechanism may be obtained. A palatal lift functions somewhat differently than the speech bulb. Its acts to elevate the soft palate and enable some degree of closure for speech.

Practitioners need to keep in mind that velopharyngeal closure for speech is a dynamic process and must remember that an intraoral view or simple perceptual screening task are not adequate for differential diagnosis. The diagnosis of a velopharyngeal deficit resulting from some type of neurologic disease or velopharyngeal insufficiency that is due to a structural impairment is based on a battery of measures that incorporate perceptual, acoustic, and physiologic data (Bzoch, 1997; Shelton & Trier, 1976; Shprintzen, 1995).

Pharynx

The pharynx—or pharyngeal cavity—plays an important role in speech, breathing, and deglutition. It is a flexible cavity that forms the upper part of both the respiratory and digestive systems. Daniloff (1973) emphasizes the significance of the pharynx in speech production and summarizes a study by Kelsey and his associates, who report variations in cavity dimension during production of various speech sounds. Similarly, Zemlin (1998) provides a succinct description of the resonating function of the pharynx and confirms that variations in cavity dimensions do occur during speech; however, he feels that major modifications in transfer function are more within the province of tongue and soft palate articulations during speech.

The pharynx is an elongated muscular tube that extends from the skull base to the inferior border of the cricoid cartilage (Zemlin, 1998). It is made up of three different bands of tissue, which include a fibrous layer known as the *pharyngeal aponeurosis*, a mucous layer, and a muscular layer. There are three pairs of constrictor muscles that make up the muscular layer. The paired muscles are the superior, middle, and inferior constrictor muscles. The superior constrictor muscle is located in the upper pharynx and plays a key role in speech production, primarily as an integral part in the valving action of velopharyngeal closure.

The pharynx is made up of the nasopharynx, oropharynx, and laryngopharynx. The oropharynx—or that part of the pharynx that extends superiorly from the level of the soft palate and inferiorly to the level of the hyoid bone—is emphasized, because it is important in speech production and can be viewed during an oral examination (Zemlin, 1998). The pharynx, nasal cavities, and oral cavity connect via the oropharyngeal isthmus; within the isthmus lies the anterior and posterior faucial pillars. Anatomically, the boundaries of the fauces embody the palatine arches or faucial pillars laterally, the soft palate superiorly, and the dorsum of the tongue inferiorly. The anterior faucial pillars consist of the paired palatoglossus muscles. Muscle contractions of this paired muscle constrict the anterior faucial arch. The palatopharyngeus muscles form the posterior faucial pillar or pharyngopalatine arch. Contractions of these paired muscles are significant in deglutition.

The palatine tonsils are located in the tonsillar fossa, a triangular space located between the anterior and posterior faucial pillars. The palatine tonsils form a portion of a ring of tonsillar tissue that encircles the oropharynx. This ring of lymphoid tissue is referred to as *Waldeyer's ring*. The palatine tonsils are located laterally, the adenoids superiorly, and the lingual tonsil inferiorly in the ring. Motor and sensory control to the pharyngeal area is achieved by the glossopharyngeal (CN IX) and vagus nerves (CN X).

The palatine tonsils are usually quite easy to observe in young individuals if the child cooperates and is not apprehensive about the examination. In some cases, the palatine tonsils are hypertrophied so that there is midline contact. The hypertrophy may have an adverse influence on speech (Spriestersbach et al., 1978). D'Antonio and Campanelli (1995) provide a cogent discussion of velopharyngeal function, and they identify possible problems that may be associated with the palatine tonsils. The authors also list a number of studies that identify hypertrophied tonsils as a causal factor in velopharyngeal insufficiency. Finkelstein et al. (1994) suggest that hypertrophic tonsils can negatively influence the resonant characteristics of the voice. Generally, hypertrophied tonsils do not hinder velopharyngeal closure, but when they extend superiorly into the oropharynx, resonance problems may occur. Practitioners need to remember that the tonsils increase in size until the client is approximately 9–12 years of age. Mason (1994) indicates that the rapid period of tonsillar growth is followed by a gradual involution of the lymphoid tissue. Nevertheless, clients with a history of lymphoid disease and infection may present with enlarged tonsils into adulthood.

Currently, fewer numbers of children undergo a tonsillectomy and adenoidectomy procedure because medical emphasis is on the protective role of these structures. Of the two, one needs to be most concerned about the adenoids for speech. The adenoids are typically situated in the concave portion of the nasopharynx and cannot be observed visually. This is the general site of contact between the soft palate and pharyngeal wall during closure activity. The adenoids gradually increase in size to puberty and then gradually begin to atrophy. At the same time of atrophy, there is an increase in the vertical distance between the soft palate and the adenoids. In some cases, clients may experience problems with velopharyngeal closure for speech after a tonsillectomy and adenoidectomy procedure because a problem such as a submucous cleft palate is unmasked.

Breathing

Breathing is critical for life support and requisite for speech production. The main function of breath support is to supply oxygen to the body and remove carbon dioxide. This process entails the transfer of air to and from special gas-exchange surfaces located in the body. Speech production without appropriate breath support and controlled exhalation would be impossible.

Hixon (1987) succinctly describes the importance of breathing in speech and suggests that the naturalness of breathing does not provide significant cues as to how vital respiration is in the speech production process. The respiratory pump is responsible for a number of functions during speech. Structures of the vocal tract are displaced, and pressures and flows are created through the valving actions of the articulators. Moreover, the pump is also an important component in the control of parameters such as loudness, pitch, stress, and the segmentation of speech into various linguistic units.

Despite the implicit importance of breathing for speech production, some investigators do not assess breathing in the oral examination (Dworkin, 1978; Emerick & Hatten, 1979 ; Mason & Simon, 1977; Spriestersbach et al., 1978). However, other investigators (Hutchinson et al., 1979; Nation & Aram, 1977; Peterson & Marquardt, 1981; Robbins & Klee, 1987) do incorporate observations of breathing. (Appendices 6C and 6D give examples of oral speech motor control protocols.) Research in respiratory function (e.g., Hixon, 1973) shows that breathing is a complex process that necessitates the use of instrumentation for accurate and reliable measurement. Hoit et al. (1993) caution that respiratory problems can affect other speech systems. For example, variations in voice onset time are often associated with problems of laryngeal coordination or upper airway articulation. However, in some clinical populations—such as those with hearing impairment or cervical spinal cord injury—there are often alternations in voice onset time that are caused by abnormal lung volumes.

The muscles of respiration are divided into muscles of inhalation and exhalation. The inhalation and exhalation phases of respiration use different muscle groups. The division of muscle groups differs further if the individual is engaged in quiet or forced breathing (Hixon, 1987; Zemlin, 1981). Zemlin (1998) makes an anatomic distinction between the inhalation muscles, which are primarily thoracic, and the muscles of exhalation, which are primarily abdominal.

The chief muscle of inspiration is the diaphragm. The diaphragm is a dome-shaped layer of muscle tissue that divides the heart and lungs inside the rib cage from the abdomen. During contraction, the diaphragm flattens out and thus allows expansion of the thorax. The abdominal muscles must be in relaxation to permit the force of the descending diaphragm to force the viscera downward and forward.

The external intercostals are muscles that are also involved in quiet inspiration (Hixon, 1973). The muscles—which are situated at the bottom of each rib obliquely and attach in an anterior direction to the top of the next lower rib—act to elevate the rib cage and increase the anterior/posterior and lateral dimensions of the rib cage. The anterior (intercartilaginous) part of the internal intercostals also plays a role in inhalation, but the bulk of the internal intercostal muscles is arranged to function primarily in exhalation. Other muscles that raise the rib cage or elongate the chest anteriorly come into play during forceful inhalation. These muscles encompass elevators from the neck, elevators and tensors from the thorax and shoulder girdle, and extensors from the back (Zemlin, 1998).

During calm exhalation, it is likely that muscular forces do not play an important role. Typically, the inclination of the stretched abdominal muscles and intercostals to return to their relaxed state and the effects of gravity in pulling down on the rib cage are adequate to diminish the volume of the thorax. During speech, contractions of the internal intercostals and abdominal muscles compress the rib cage and force the diaphragm upward. Vigorous exhalation often brings other thoracic muscles into contraction that flex the spine forward, lower the shoulders, and further lower the rib cage (Hixon, 1973; Zemlin, 1987).

There are differences between the inhalation/exhalation cycle necessary for life support and regulation of breath control during speech. In speech, inhalation is shortened and the exhalation cycle is increased to generate sufficient air pressure and flow for voice, articulation, and resonance. Note that the contribution of specific muscles varies significantly along the continuum of quiet breathing to isolated vowel production, to conversational speech, and finally to shouting. Moreover, other extreme conditions of muscle contraction that can influence aerodynamic control during speech include the moment-to-moment breathing rate when altered by factors like physical exertion, psychological fatigue, and body posture. These factors make it unfeasible to distinguish particular breathing postures (such as "abdominal" or "thoracic") and which postures do—or should—predominate for speech. Motor innervation to the lungs and diaphragm is provided by branches of the vagus nerve (CN X).

Breath control for some clients is a problem, and it is possible that speech or voice is negatively affected. For example, normal respiratory patterns may become disturbed in persons with histories of vocal abuse. The affected individual may frequently engage in inhaling and exhaling air more forcefully than necessary, ending in long-term physical abuse to the vocal folds (Boone & McFarlane, 1987). Frequently, stutterers develop atypical strategies for regulating breathing during moments of stuttering (St. Louis, 1979).

Clavicular breathing is a breathing pattern that has been described in the literature and remains highly controversial. Clavicular breathing is a lifting of the shoulders during inhalation—a normal strategy in strenuous inhalation when the body needs increased amounts of oxygen. When the shoulders are raised, the volume of the thorax and consequent lung volume is enlarged. If shoulder elevation occurs during quiet breathing or speech breathing, it may be an indicator that the person is not allowing the diaphragm to move downward adequately. Rather, the individual contracts the stomach musculature and hampers the regular anterior extension of the abdomen (Boone, 1977). Some speakers use clavicular breathing postures to sustain the semblance of a compact waist and large chest (Hixon, 1975). The shoulders must be raised if the diaphragm cannot efficiently increase the thoracic volumes necessary for normal inhalation. Zemlin (1998) indicates that increased use of the neck muscles during breathing is symptomatic of persons with chronic lung disease.

Duffy (1995) identifies a number of concerns that need to be taken into account when examining the respiratory patterns of persons who may possibly have neurologic disease. Clients should be examined at rest to examine body posture. If body posture is not normal, the client should be questioned in regard to problems with respiration like shortness of breath at rest or during some form of physical exertion. Breathing rate should also be examined for irregular patterns that may correlate with sudden or decreased movement of the abdominal or thoracic areas.

Hixon and his research group (1982) report a relatively easy procedure that may be used to estimate the capacity of a client to create subglottal air pressure adequate for speech production. The patient is instructed to blow into a straw that is suspended in water to a specified depth. Research by Netsell and Hixon (1978) shows that the minimal requirement for speech production would be the continuous generation of air pressure at 5 cm H_2O for a period of 5 seconds. There are other instrumentation and measurement procedures that provide quantitative measures of respiration, and the reader is referred to some excellent texts on the subject (Baken, 1987; Kent, 1994).

The presence or absence of mouth breathing during silent periods is an observation that is made usually on all current examination protocols. Habitual mouth breathing is frequently a significant clue to various types of nasal or nasopharyngeal obstruction, like hypertrophied tonsils or adenoids, deviated nasal septum, chronic upper respiratory infection, midface growth deficiency, or surgical intervention (Bardach, 1995; Dworkin, 1978; Jung, 1989). Such a diagnosis should be considered only after careful observation of the client, because the open-mouth posture may not be a symptom of a breathing problem but a habit formed from a past problem that has resolved (Kellum, 1994).

Functional Movements of the Articulators

As part of the oral mechanism examination, clients generally engage in various oral motor movement tasks that include nonspeech and speech stimuli. The rationale is to obtain a measure of the integrity of the neuromotor system. Perusal of the literature indicates numerous tasks that may be used to assess motor behavior (Sonies et al., 1987). For example, Kent (1994) includes a number of formal and informal measures that assess structure and function of the oral mechanism. Tasks such as puffing the cheeks with air, positioning the tongue in certain ways, and opening the mouth in the presence of resistance to the jaw are examples of maneuvers that are commonly used. There are also measures that provide quantitative measures of muscular variables, such as strength and endurance. For example, Robin et al. (1992) use an air-filled bulb that is inserted in the oral cavity. The client is instructed to squeeze the bulb with the tongue. The tongue pressure creates a pressure differential that is measured and displayed on a digital readout.

Diadochokinesis, which is the rapid repetitive movement of a muscular structure, has an extensive history in the speech-language pathology literature for examining motor skill, coordination, and neuromotor integration (Duffy, 1995). A number of diagnostic texts and examinations suggest that maximum diadochokinetic rates for nonsense syllables like /pʌ/, /tʌ/, and /kʌ/ and multisyllable sequences like /pʌtʌ/ or /pʌtʌkʌ/ be used in the examination (Emerick & Hatten, 1979; Hutchinson et al., 1979; Mason & Simon, 1977; Mason et al., 1988; Nation & Aram, 1977; Peterson & Marquardt, 1981; Spriestersbach et al., 1978; St. Louis & Ruscello, 2000).

Spriestersbach et al. (1978) summarize a series of studies that examine diadochokinesis and conclude that slower-than-expected diadochokinetic rates may have some degree of diagnostic importance for the practitioner. In summarizing the literature, they report that the average child produces between three and six repetitions per second for /pʌ/; 3–5½ repetitions per second for /tʌ/; and 3–5 repetitions per second for /kʌ/. Fletcher's (1972) normative data for elementary school children between 6 and 10 years of age agree with the figures for repetitions of single syllables, but the guidelines for /pʌtʌkʌ/ are somewhat ambiguous. For example, Yoss and Darley (1974) and Leshkin (1948) find average repetition rates for children of approximately three to four repetitions per second, whereas Robinson (1973) and Fletcher (1972) report repetition rates of 1–1½ repetitions per second for the task.

Slower-than-average diadochokinesis is reported for a variety of speech-language disorders, but the data are equivocal. Winitz (1969) feels that past history of a phonological disorder could account for a difference between comparisons of normal speakers and children with phonological disorders. He concludes that there is no significant support for the position that children with phonological disorders exhibit slower-than-average diadochokinetic rates. Contrary to the Winitz study, Dworkin (1978) and Yoss and Darley (1974) find differences between normal children and children with moderate to severe phonological disorders and mild problems such as lisping.

St. Louis and Ruscello (2000) present diadochokinetic data from a large group of normal speakers ranging in age from approximately 5 years to 77 years. The data show repetition times that are quite similar from age 8 through adulthood. Single syllable repetition rates (pʌ, tʌ, kʌ) average approximately five to six per second, disyllables (pʌtʌ) approximately four per second, and trisyllables (pʌtʌkʌ) approximately two per second.

Weismer (1997) critically discusses the role of oral motor diagnostic procedures in the evaluation of speech disorders and concludes that diadochokinetic rates may not furnish important diagnostic data. The author suggests that diadochokinetic tasks are quasispeech tasks because they do not simulate speech production. The rapid repetition of speech stimuli is not consistent with speaking rates and articulatory trajectories found in conversational speech. Moreover, Kent et al. (1987) survey the literature on maximum speech performance tasks, such as diadochokinesis, and discuss a number of shortcomings with the data. (Appendix 6E is a table of normative syllable repetition rates from this study.) The authors first state that there is a great deal of inter- and intrasubject variability in the performance data reported across studies reviewed. Second, the requirements of normal speech production are within the parameters established by the measures of maximum performance. Third, maximum performance tasks have a long tradition in the speech-language pathology literature, but the normative database is limited across the life span. As a consequence, the practitioner should use maximum speech performance tests carefully with clients and interpret the results with caution.

Commercial Tests

Dworkin-Culatta Oral Mechanism Examination and Treatment System
The Dworkin-Culatta Oral Mechanism Examination and Treatment System (D-COME; Dworkin & Culatta, 1996) was designed for the differential diagnosis and treatment of motor speech and orofacial structural disorders. The test materials consist of a screening test and deep tests. The

screening test requires approximately 10 minutes to administer and evaluates oral structures and functions across eight diagnostic areas. If a client fails the screening, the deep tests are administered for a more in-depth examination of the eight diagnostic areas so that a differential diagnosis may be established. The diagnostic areas include

1.   Facial status
2.   Lip functioning
3.   Jaw functioning
4.   Hard palate status
5.   Tongue functioning
6.   Velopharyngeal functioning
7.   Dental and gingival status
8.   Motor speech programming abilities

The D-COME tests may be used with young children through adults. The items on the screening test are scored as either "Yes" (a problem was identified) or "No" (a problem was not identified). The deep tests are scored by using a check [√] to indicate normal performance and a 3-point numeric scale to rate abnormal behavior. An abnormally appearing structure or function may be rated 1 (a mild impairment), 2 (a moderate impairment), and 3 (a severe impairment). The manual contains extensive information regarding diagnostic symptoms and differential diagnosis of various motor speech disorders, such as dysarthria, and structural disorders, such as cleft palate. There is also a comprehensive section of therapy intervention that is based on the differential diagnosis results. The D-COME is not a standardized test that includes normative performance data or reliability or validity information. It is a clinical tool that allows screening or in-depth examination, and it may be used in formulating a clinical diagnosis and a treatment strategy.

Frenchay Dysarthria Assessment

The Frenchay Dysarthria Assessment (Enderby, 1983) is an orofacial test used in the differential diagnosis of the dysarthrias. The test has 11 different categories that are evaluated firsthand or obtained through history information concerning factors that are associated with the disorder. The categories of assessment are *reflex, respiration, lips, jaw, palate, laryngeal, tongue, intelligibility, rate, sensation,* and *associated factors*. Evaluation items are rated along a 9-point rating scale that ranges from no problem to a severe problem. The scoring form is designed to display a profile of abilities that can be used to identify strengths and weaknesses. In addition, the manual provides profiles of subjects with different dysarthrias so that the performance of a particular client may be compared for diagnostic purposes.

The test is used for clients who are suspect of having dysarthria. It is used specifically for adult subjects, but it could be used with school-age clients. Interjudge reliability and validity studies were carried out and are reported in the manual. The test is a comprehensive instrument with specific administration instructions and scoring categories.

Oral Speech Mechanism Screening Examination

The Oral Speech Mechanism Screening Examination (3rd ed.) (OSMSE-3; St. Louis & Ruscello, 2000) is a screening test that may be used with clients undergoing diagnosis for speech, language, and related disorders. OSMSE-3 is organized to permit a rapid examination of the orofacial complex. Structure and function observations of the lips, tongue, jaws, teeth, hard palate, soft palate, pharynx, breathing, and speech motor control are made using a two-category scoring system. The scoring category depends on the specific item being assessed. For example, some items are marked [+] for no deviation and [–] for a deviation, whereas others provide a set of choices that require a [√] to identify the appropriate category among a set of responses. There is a scoring form that is used to record all client responses. Separate structure, function, and total scores are calculated to permit normative comparison.

The OSMSE-3 may be used with clients from 5 years of age through adulthood. Reliability and validity data are reported for the test, along with test results of different groups of speech-disordered subjects. The manual includes detailed instructions for administering the test, and there is information pertaining to the growth and development of the orofacial complex. There is also an interpretation section that discusses potential problems in structure and function that the practitioner may refer to during an assessment.

Test of Oral Structures and Functions

The underlying rationale of the Test of Oral Structures and Functions (TOSF; Vitali, 1995) is that a client exhibits performance differences that enable etiologic classification into functional, neurologic, and structural disorder types. There are five subtests, which include

1. Speech survey
2. Verbal oral functioning
3. Nonverbal oral functions
4. Orofacial structures
5. History-behavioral survey

The speech survey consists of an assessment of articulation, rate/prosody, fluency, and voice in a conversational sample that may be a spontaneous or elicited speech sample. The speech production parameters of resonance balance, articulatory precision, and rate/prosody are examined in the verbal oral functioning subtest. Nonverbal oral functions—such as individual and sequential volitional and nonvolitional movements—are assessed in the nonverbal oral functions subtest. The orofacial structures subtest allows observation of the oral structures, and the history-behavioral survey subtest contains a series of questions pertaining to the development and maintenance of the communication disorder.

The TOSF may be used with clients from age 7 through adulthood. Client performance on individual items is scored as normal, inconsistent, or consistent error performance. The only exception is the history-behavioral survey subtest, which is not included in the scoring conventions but is a history-gathering instrument. The raw score subtest totals are determined and the resultant scores converted to scaled scores. The scaled scores are then compared with cutoff scores that correspond to the categories of unremarkable, borderline, impaired, and marked impairment. The manual contains TOSF performance patterns of subjects who have various communication disorders, such as dysarthria. Validity and reliability data are reported for the test.

Verbal Motor Production Assessment for Children

The Verbal Motor Production Assessment for Children (Hayden & Square, 1999) is an instrument designed to examine the motor speech system of children who present with speech production problems. The authors indicate that it can be used to distinguish between children with motor speech disorders and children who do not have such an etiologic base to their articulatory/phonological disorder. In addition, test performance patterns can also be used to differentiate developmental apraxia from developmental dysarthrias and identify potential input modalities for use in treatment. The assessment stimuli consist of reflex behavior and vegetative and volitional nonspeech and speech items. The speech items include both meaningful and nonmeaningful linguistic stimuli. The primary subtest areas are *global motor control, focal oromotor control,* and *sequencing.* Two supplemental areas, *connected speech* and *language control and speech characteristics,* are also part of the examination.

The test is appropriate for children from 3 to 12 years of age. Scoring alternatives depend on the particular item that is being evaluated. The test booklet contains extensive administration information and scoring directions for the examiner. The authors have also developed a videotape that provides various administration and scoring examples. Raw scores are converted into percent scores and may be compared with normative comparison data. The normative data are based on the responses of a large test group. Reliability and validity data are reported for the test, along with test results of various groups of subjects with articulatory/phonological disorders. The manual contains case history illustrations and recommendations for intervention.

Oral Motor Tests

Bedside Evaluation of Dysphagia

The Bedside Evaluation of Dysphagia (Hardy, 1995) is an assessment protocol for the behavioral examination of clients with dysphagia. The protocol consists of separate sections that provide information on *behavioral characteristics, cognition and communication screening, oral-motor examination,* and *oral-pharyngeal dysphagia symptoms assessment.* The oral-motor examination contains items that evaluate the sensory and motor status of the lips, tongue, soft palate, cheeks, mandible, and larynx. Client responses are judged as either within normal limits or impaired. The manual includes an in-depth section that describes each test item and responses that would be considered within normal limits or impaired.

The Bedside Evaluation of Dysphagia is designed for adult clients who are suspect of having dysphagia. It is not a formal test that has been subject to standardization, but an assessment protocol that may be used by practitioners who treat adult clients with dysphagia.

Establishing Dysphagia Programs: A Guide for Speech-Language Pathologists

Establishing Dysphagia Programs: A Guide for Speech-Language Pathologists (Rehab Choice Inc., 1993) is a program that was developed for use with clients who have dysphagia. The manual provides information on topics that range from behavioral assessment to swallowing to treatment strategies to information for attending physicians. For some topics, there are reproducible forms for use. The evaluation of structure and function of peripheral speech and swallowing mechanism is used to evaluate the oral mechanism in a systematic fashion. There are individual sections for observing the oral structures at rest and during movement. The lips, teeth, tongue, cheeks, floor of the mouth, hard palate, soft palate, uvula, faucial arches, and posterior pharyngeal wall are evaluated. Scoring conventions for structure and function are included for use by the practitioner.

Establishing Dysphagia Programs: A Guide for Speech-Language Pathologists is a clinical tool for the overall assessment and treatment of adult clients who have dysphagia. It is not a standardized test. A subsection does furnish data on oral-motor performance.

Program for the Assessment and Instruction of Swallowing

The Program for the Assessment and Instruction of Swallowing (Mulfeter & Rosenfield, 1993) is a program that was developed for the assessment and treatment of clients with dysphagia. There are separate protocols for the behavioral examination of dysphagia (*clinical evaluation of swallowing*), instrumental assessment of dysphagia (*modified barium swallow study*), and implementation of a dysphagia treatment program (*swallowing instruction protocol*). The clinical evaluation of swallowing contains an oral screening section that examines the structure and function of the oral mechanism. Assessment items include dentition, dentures, dry swallow, uvula and soft palate, velopharyngeal closure, laryngeal function, muscle tone, abnormal reflexes, orofacial movements, oral apraxia, and sensation. Each assessment item is scored according to the information desired for that particular structure or function. For example, velopharyngeal closure can be rated as hypernasal, normal, or hyponasal.

The Program for the Assessment and Instruction of Swallowing is a program for the assessment and treatment of adult clients who have dysphagia. It has not been subject to standardization as an actual test would be. A subtest of the clinical evaluation of swallowing is designed to examine the oral mechanism.

Rehabilitation Institute of Chicago Clinical Evaluation of Dysphagia

The Clinical Evaluation of Dysphagia (Cherney et al., 1986) is an evaluation tool for conducting a behavioral assessment of dysphagia, and it serves as a recording instrument for both behavioral and instrumental assessments. The data on oral structure and function are recorded on an evaluation sheet. The observations of structure and function are made while the person is given various consistencies of food. The lips, tongue, mandible, velopharyngeal mechanism, and pharynx are studied. In some cases, the practitioner rates performance as "adequate-inadequate" or checks a performance dimension according to response alternatives included on the evaluation.

As with many other tools in the area of swallowing disorders, the oral mechanism examination is just one aspect of the evaluation protocol. The Clinical Evaluation of Dysphagia is not a standardized test, but it may be used with adults who have dysphagia.

References

American Speech-Language Hearing Association. (1990). *Report update: AIDS/HIV: Implications for speech-language pathologists and audiologists. ASHA, 32,* 46–48.

American Speech-Language Hearing Association. (1991a). The role of the speech-language pathologist in the management of oral myofunctional disorders. *ASHA, 33,* (Suppl. 5), 7.

American Speech-Language Hearing Association. (1991b). Chronic communicable diseases and risk management in the schools. *Language, Speech, and Hearing Services in the Schools, 22,* 345–352.

American Speech-Language Hearing Association. (1993). Orofacial myofunctional disorders: Knowledge and skills. *ASHA, 35,* (Suppl. 10), 21–23.

Angle, E. (1907). *Malocclusion of the teeth* (7th ed.). Philadelphia: S. S. White Dental Mfg. Co.

Aronson, A. E. (1980). Dysarthria. In T. J. Hixon, L. D. Shriberg, & J. H. Saxman (Eds.), *Introduction to communicative disorders* (pp. 407–447). Englewood Cliffs, NJ: Prentice-Hall.

Baken, R. J. (1987). *Clinical measurement of speech and voice.* San Diego: College-Hill Press.

Bankson, N. W., & Byrne, M. C. (1962). The relationship between missing teeth and selected consonant sounds. *Journal of Speech and Hearing Disorders, 27,* 341–348.

Bardach, J. (1995). Secondary surgery for velopharyngeal insufficiency. In R. J. Shprintzen & J. Bardach (Eds.), *Cleft palate speech management* (pp. 277–294). St. Louis: Mosby.

Bardach, J., & Salyer, K. E. (1995). Cleft palate repair: Anatomy, timing, goals, principles, and techniques. In R. J. Shprintzen & J. Bardach (Eds.), *Cleft palate speech management* (pp. 102–136). St. Louis: Mosby.

Bloomer H. H. (1971). Speech defects associated with dental malocclusions and related abnormalities. In L. E. Travis (Ed.), *Handbook of speech pathology and audiology* (pp. 713–766). New York: Meredith.

Boone, D. R. (1977). *The voice and voice therapy* (2nd ed.). Englewood Cliffs, NJ: Prentice-Hall.

Boone, D. R., & McFarlane, S. C. (1987). *The voice and voice therapy* (4th ed.). Englewood Cliffs, NJ: Prentice-Hall.

Bosma, J. F. (1976). Sensorimotor examination of the mouth and pharynx. *Frontiers in Oral Physiology, 2,* 78–107.

Bradley, D. P. (1997). Congenital and acquired velopharyngeal inadequacy. In K. R. Bzoch (Ed.), *Communicative disorders related to cleft lip and palate* (4th ed.) (pp. 223–244). Austin, TX: Pro-Ed.

Brescia, N .J. (1971). Anatomy of the lip and palate. In W. C. Grabb, S. W. Rosenstein, & K. R. Bzoch (Eds.), *Cleft lip and palate: Surgical, dental, and speech aspect* (pp. 3–20). Boston: Little, Brown.

Bzoch, K. R. (1997). Clinical assessment, evaluation, and management of 11 categorical aspects of cleft palate speech disorders. In K. R. Bzoch (Ed.), *Communicative disorders related to cleft lip and palate* (4th ed.) (pp. 261–312). Austin, TX: Pro-Ed.

Carey, J. C., Stevens, C. A., & Haskins, R. (1992). Craniofacial malformations and their syndromes: An overview for the speech and hearing practitioner. *Clinics in Communication Disorders, 2,* 58–72.

Caruso, A. J., & Strand, E. A. *Clinical management of motor speech disorders in children.* New York: Thieme.

Cassell, M. D., & Elkadi, H. (1995). Anatomy and physiology of the palate and velopharyngeal structures. In R. J. Shprintzen & J. Bardach (Eds.), *Cleft palate speech management* (pp. 45–62). St. Louis: Mosby.

Cherney, L. R., Cantieri, C. A., & Pannell, J. J. (1986). *Clinical evaluation of dysphagia.* Rockville, MD: Aspen Publishers.

Coston, G. N., Sayetta, R. B., Friedman, H. I., Weinrich, M. C., Macera, C. A., Meeks, K., McAndrews, S. K., & Morales, K. S. (1992). Craniofacial screening profile: Quick screening for congenital malformations. *Cleft Palate-Craniofacial Journal, 29,* 87–91.

Daniloff, R. G. (1973). Normal articulation processes. In F. D. Minifie, T. J. Hixon, & F. Williams (Eds.), *Normal aspects of speech, hearing, and language* (pp. 169–210). Englewood Cliffs, NJ: Prentice-Hall.

D'Antonio, L. L., & Campanelli, J. (1995). Velopharyngeal function. *Otolaryngology and Head and Neck Surgery, 3,* 157–163.

Darley, F. L. (1978). Differential diagnosis of acquired motor speech disorders. In F. L. Darley & D. C. Spriestersbach (Eds.), *Diagnostic methods in speech pathology* (pp. 492–513). New York: Harper & Row.

Darley, F. L., Aronson, A. E., & Brown, J. R. (1975). *Motor speech disorders.* Philadelphia: W. B. Saunders.

Duffy, J. R. (1995). *Motor speech disorders.* St. Louis: Mosby.

Dworkin, J. P. (1978). Differential diagnosis of motor speech disorders: The clinical examination of the speech mechanism. *Journal of the National Student Speech and Hearing Association, 6,* 37–62.

Dworkin, J. P., & Culatta, R. A. (1996). *Dworkin-Culatta oral mechanism examination and treatment system.* Farmington Hills, MI: Edgewood Press.

Emerick, L.L. & Hatten, J.H. (1979). *Diagnosis and evaluation in speech pathology* (2nd ed.). Englewood Cliffs, NJ: Prentice-Hall.

Enderby, P. M. (1983). *Frenchay dysarthria assessment.* Austin, TX: Pro-Ed.

Ewanowski, S. J., & Saxman, J. H. (1980). Orofacial disorders. In T. J. Hixon, L. D. Shriberg, & J. H. Saxman (Eds.), *Introduction to communication disorders* (pp. 352–405). Englewood Cliffs, NJ: Prentice-Hall.

Ferketic, M. M., & Gardner, K. (1994). *Orofacial myology: Beyond tongue thrust.* Rockville, MD: American Speech-Language Hearing Association.

Finkelstein, Y., Nachmani, A., & Ophir, D. (1994). The functional role of the tonsils in speech. *Archives of Otolaryngology and Head and Neck Surgery, 120,* 846–851.

Fletcher, S. G. (1972). Time-by-count measurement of diadochokinetic syllable rate. *Journal of Speech and Hearing Research, 15,* 763–770.

Fletcher, S. G., & Meldrum, J. R. (1968). Lingual function and relative length of the lingual frenulum. *Journal of Speech and Hearing Research, 11,* 382–390.

Fox, D., & Johns, D. (1970). Predicting velopharyngeal closure with a modified tongue-anchor technique. *Journal of Speech and Hearing Disorders, 35,* 248–251.

Fritzell, B. (1969). The velopharyngeal muscles in speech: An electromyographic and cineradiographic study. *Acta Otolaryngologica, 250* (Supplement), 1–81.

Hale, S. T., Kellum, G. D., Richardson, J. F., Messer, S. C., Gross, A. M., & Sisakun, S. (1992). Oral motor control, posturing, and myofunctional variables in 8-year-olds. *Journal of Speech and Hearing Research, 35,* 1203–1208.

Hardy, E. (1995). *Bedside evaluation of dysphagia.* Bisbee, AZ: Imaginart.

Hayden, D., & Square, P. (1999). *Verbal motor production assessment for children.* San Antonio, TX: Psychological Corporation.

Hixon, T. J. (1973). Respiratory function in speech. In F. D. Minifie, T. J. Hixon, & F. Williams (Eds.), *Normal aspects of speech, hearing and language* (pp. 73–125). San Diego: College-Hill Press.

Hixon, T. J. (1975). Anatomy for speech. Short course presented at the New York Speech and Hearing Association Convention, Liberty, NY.

Hixon, T. J. (1987). Respiratory function in speech. In T. J. Hixon (Ed.), *Respiratory function in speech and song* (pp. 1–54). San Diego: College-Hill Press.

Hixon, T. J., & Abbs, J. H. (1980). Normal speech production. In T. J. Hixon, L. D. Shriberg, & J. H. Saxman (Eds.), *Introduction to communication disorders* (pp. 43–87). Englewood Cliffs, NJ: Prentice-Hall.

Hixon, T. J., Hawley, J. L., & Wilson, K. J. (1982). An around-the-house device for the clinical determination of respiratory driving pressure: A note on making simple even simpler. *Journal of Speech and Hearing Disorders, 47,* 413–415.

Hoit, J. D., Solomon, N. P., & Hixon, T. J. (1993). Effect of lung volume on voice onset time (VOT). *Journal of Speech and Hearing Research, 36,* 516–520.

Hutchinson, B. B., Hanson, M. L., & Mecham, M. J. (1979). *Diagnostic handbook of speech pathology.* Baltimore: Williams & Wilkins.

Johnson, H., & Scott, A. (1993). *A practical approach to saliva control.* Tucson, AZ: Communication Skill Builders.

Jung, J. H. (1989). *Genetic syndromes in communicative disorders.* Boston/Toronto: College-Hill Press.

Kaplin, H. M. (1971). *Anatomy and physiology of speech* (2nd ed.). New York: McGraw-Hill.

Kellum, G. D. (1994). Overview of oral myology. In M. M. Ferketic & K. Gardner (Eds.), *Orofacial myology: Beyond tongue thrust* (pp. 1–10). Rockville, MD: American Speech-Language Hearing Association.

Kent., R. D. (1994). *Reference manual for communicative sciences and disorders: Speech and language.* Austin, TX: Pro-Ed.

Kent, R. D., Kent, J. F., & Rosenbeck, J. C. (1987). Maximum performance tests of speech production. *Journal of Speech and Hearing Disorders, 52,* 367–387.

Keuhn, D. P. (1982). Assessment of resonance disorders. In Lass, N. J., McReynolds, L. V., Northern, J. L., & Yoder, D. E. (Eds.), *Speech, language and hearing* (pp. 499–525). Philadelphia: W. B. Saunders.

Kier, W. M., & Smith, K. K. (1985). Tongues, tentacles and trunks: The biomechanics of movement in muscular-hydrostats. *Zoological Journal of the Linnean Society, 83,* 307–324.

LaPointe, L. L., & Wertz, R. T. (1974). Oral movement abilities and articulatory characteristics of brain injured adults. *Perceptual and Motor Skills,* 39–46.

Leeper, H. A., Sills, P. S., & Charles, D. H. (1993). Prosthodontic management of maxillofacial and palatal defects. In K. T. Moller & C. D. Starr (Eds.), *Cleft palate* (pp. 145–188). Austin, TX: Pro-Ed.

Leshkin, S. (1948). *A study of diadochokinetic movements of lips and tongues in children.* Unpublished master's thesis, University of Michigan.

Logemann, J. A. (1983). *Evaluation and treatment of swallowing disorders.* Austin, TX: Pro-Ed.

Logemann, J. A. (1998). *Evaluation and treatment of swallowing disorders* (2nd ed.). Austin, TX: Pro-Ed.

Love, R. J. (1992). *Childhood motor speech disability.* New York: Macmillan.

Luchsinger, R., & Arnold, G. E. (1965). *Voice-speech-language clinical communicology: Its physiology and pathology.* Belmont, CA: Wadsworth.

MacKay, J. R. A. (1978). *Introducing practical phonetics.* Boston: Little, Brown.

Mason, R. M. (1994). Basic medical-dental considerations. In M. M. Ferketic & K. Gardner (Eds.), *Orofacial myology: Beyond tongue thrust* (pp. 11–20). Rockville, MD: American Speech-Language Hearing Association.

Mason, R. M., & Proffit, W. R. (1974). The tongue thrust controversy: Background and recommendations. *Journal of Speech and Hearing Disorders, 30,* 115–132.

Mason, R. M., & Simon, C. (1977). An orofacial examination checklist. *Language, Speech, and Hearing Services in the Schools, 8,* 155–163.

Mason R. M., Peterson-Falzone, S. J., Sonies, B., & Webster, D. B. (1988). *Evaluation of the speech and swallowing mechanisms.* ASHA Video Conference. Rockville, MD.

McMillan, M. O., & Willette, S. J. (1988). Aseptic technique: A procedure for preventing disease transmission in the practice environment. *ASHA, 30,* 35–38.

McWilliams, B. J., Morris, H. L., & Shelton, R. L. (1990). *Cleft palate speech* (2nd ed.). Philadelphia: B. C. Decker.

Moon, J., & Kuehn, D. (1996). Anatomy and physiology of normal and disordered velopharyngeal function for speech. *NCVS Status and Progress Report, 9,* 143–158.

Moon, J., & Kuehn, D. (1997). Anatomy and physiology of normal and disordered velopharyngeal function for speech. In K. R. Bzoch (Ed.), *Communicative disorders related to cleft lip and palate* (4th ed.) (pp. 45–68). Austin, TX: Pro-Ed.

Mulfeter, V. A., & Rosenfield, J. F. (1993). *Program for the assessment and instruction of swallowing.* Vero Beach, FL: Speech Bin.

Nation, J. E., & Aram, D. M. (1977). *Diagnosis of speech and language disorders.* St. Louis: Mosby.

Netsell, R., & Hixon, T. J. (1978). A noninvasive method for clinically estimating subglottal air pressure. *Journal of Speech and Hearing Disorders, 43,* 326–330.

Perkins, W. H., & Kent, R. D. (1986). *Functional anatomy of speech, language, and hearing.* San Diego: College Hill Press, Inc.

Perlman, A. L., & Christensen, J. (1997). Topography and functional anatomy of the swallowing structures. In A. D. Perlman & K. Schulze-Delrieu (Eds.), *Deglutition and its management* (pp. 15–42). San Diego: Singular Publishing Group, Inc.

Perlman, A. L., Lu, C., & Jones, B. (1997). Radiographic contrast examination of the mouth, pharynx, and esophagus. In A. D. Perlman & K. Schulze-Delrieu (Eds.), *Deglutition and its management* (pp. 153–200). San Diego: Singular Publishing Group, Inc.

Peterson, H. A., & Marquardt, T. P. (1981). *Appraisal and diagnosis of speech and language disorders.* Englewood Cliffs, NJ: Prentice-Hall.

Peterson-Falzone, S. J. (1982). Articulation disorders in orofacial anomalies. In Lass, N. J., McReynolds, L. V., Northern, J. L., & Yoder, D. E. (Eds.), *Speech, language and hearing* (pp. 611–637). Philadelphia: W. B. Saunders.

Peterson-Falzone, S. J. (1987). Speech disorders related to craniofacial structural defects: Part 2. In Lass, N. J., McReynolds, L. V., Northern, J. L., & Yoder, D. E. (Eds.), *Handbook of speech-language pathology and audiology* (pp. 477–547). Toronto: Decker.

Rehab Choice Inc. (1993). *Establishing dysphagia programs: A guide for speech-language pathologists.* Vero Beach, FL: Speech Bin.

Robbins, J., & Klee, T. (1987). Clinical assessment of oropharyngeal motor development in young children. *Journal of Speech and Hearing Disorders, 52,* 271–277.

Robin, D. A., Goel, A., Somodi, L. B., & Luschei, E. S. (1992). Tongue strength and endurance: Relation to highly skilled movements. *Journal of Speech and Hearing Research, 35,* 1239–1245.

Robinson, K. (1973). *Development of norms for a motor examination of speech.* Unpublished master's thesis, Illinois State University.

Rosen, M. S., & Bzoch, K. R. (1997). Prosthodontic management of the individual with cleft lip and palate for speech habilitation needs. In K. R. Bzoch (Ed.), *Communicative disorders related to cleft lip and palate* (4th ed.) (pp. 153–168). Austin, TX: Pro-Ed.

Ruscello, D. M. (1997). Considerations for behavioral treatment of velopharyngeal closure for speech. In K. R. Bzoch (Ed.), *Communicative disorders related to cleft lip and palate* (4th ed.) (pp. 509–528). Austin, TX: Pro-Ed.

Ruscello, D. M., Tekieli-Koay, M. E., & Van Sickels, J. E. (1985). Speech production before and after orthognathic surgery: A review. *Oral Surgery, Oral Medicine, and Oral Pathology, 8,* 33–38.

Seagle, M. B. (1997). Primary surgical correction of cleft palate. In K. R. Bzoch (Ed.), *Communicative disorders related to cleft lip and palate* (4th ed.) (pp. 115–120). Austin, TX: Pro-Ed.

Shelton, R. L., & Trier, W. C. (1976). Issues involved in the evaluation of velopharyngeal closure. *Cleft Palate Journal, 13,* 127–137.

Shprintzen, R. J. (1995). Instrumental assessment of velopharyngeal valving. In R. J. Shprintzen & J. Bardach (Eds.), *Cleft palate speech management* (pp. 221–256). St. Louis: Mosby.

Shprintzen, R. J. (1997). *Genetic syndromes and communication disorders.* San Diego: Singular Publishing Group, Inc.

Shprintzen, R. J. (2000). *Syndrome identification for speech-language pathology.* San Diego: Singular Publishing Group, Thomson Learning.

Shprintzen, R. J., & Witzel, M. A. (1993). *Reference guide: Delineation and diagnosis of craniofacial syndromes: Effect on case management.* Rockville, MD: American Speech-Language Hearing Association.

Sicher, H., & DuBrul, E. L. (1975). *Oral anatomy* (6th ed.). St. Louis: Mosby.

Snow, K. (1961). Articulation proficiency in relation to certain dental abnormalities. *Journal of Speech and Hearing Disorders, 26,* 209–212.

Sonies, B. C., Weiffenbach, J., Atkinson, J. C., Brahim, J. Macynski, R. N., & Fox, P. C. (1987). Clinical examination of motor and sensory functions of the adult oral cavity. *Dysphagia, 1,* 178–186.

Spriestersbach, D. C., Moll, K. L., & Morris, H. L. (1961). Subject classification and articulation of speakers with cleft palates. *Journal of Speech and Hearing Research, 4,* 362–372.

Spriestersbach, D. C., Morris, H. L., & Darley, F. L. (1978). Examination of the speech mechanism. In F. L. Darley & D. C. Spriestersbach (Eds.), *Diagnostic methods in speech pathology* (2nd ed.) (pp. 322–345). New York: Harper & Row.

Starr, C. D. (1971). Dental and occlusal hazards to normal speech production. In W. C. Grabb, S. W. Rosenstein, & K. R. Bzoch (Eds.), *Cleft lip and palate: Surgical, dental, and speech aspects* (pp. 670–680). Boston: Little, Brown.

St. Louis, K. O. (1979). Linguistic and motor aspects of stuttering. In N. J. Lass (Ed.), *Speech and language: Advances in basic research and practice* (pp. 90–210). New York: Academic Press.

St. Louis, K. O., & Ruscello, D. M. (2000). *Oral speech mechanism screening examination (OSMSE)* (revised ed.). Austin, TX: Pro-Ed.

Trost-Cardamone, J. E. (1995). Diagnosis and management of speakers with craniofacial anomalies. Short course presented at the Annual Convention of the American Speech-Language Hearing Association. Orlando.

Vitali, G. J. *Test of oral structures and functions.* (1995). East Aurora, NY: Slosson Educational Publications.

Warden, P. J. (1991). Ankyloglossia: A review of the literature. *General Dentistry, 39,* 252–253.

Weismer, G. (1997). *Assessment of oromotor, nonspeech gestures in speech-language pathology: A critical review.* Telerounds presentation of the National Center for Neurogenic Communication Disorders, University of Arizona, Tucson.

Williams, W. N., & Waldron, C. M. (1985). Assessment of lingual function when ankyloglossia (tongue-tie) is suspected. *Journal of the American Dental Association, 110,* 353–356.

Wilson-Pauwels, L., Akesson, E. J., & Stewart, P. A. (1988). *Cranial nerves.* Toronto: Decker.

Winitz, H. (1969). *Articulatory acquisition and behavior.* New York: Meredith.

Witzel, M. A. (1995). Communicative impairment associated with clefting. In R. J. Shprintzen & J. Bardach (Eds.), *Cleft palate speech management* (pp. 137–166). St. Louis: Mosby.

Yorkston, K. M., Beukelman, D. R., Strand, E. A., & Bell, K. R. (1999). *Management of motor speech disorders in children and adults* (2nd ed.). Austin, TX: Pro-Ed.

Yoss, K. E., & Darley, F. L. (1974). Developmental apraxia of speech in children with defective articulation. *Journal of Speech and Hearing Research, 17,* 39–47.

Zemlin, W. R. (1981). *Speech and hearing science: Anatomy and physiology* (2nd ed.). Englewood Cliffs, NJ: Prentice-Hall.

Zemlin, W. R. (1987). *Speech and hearing science: Anatomy and physiology* (3rd ed.). Englewood Cliffs, NJ: Prentice-Hall.

Zemlin, W. R. (1998). *Speech and hearing science: Anatomy and physiology* (4th ed.). Englewood Cliffs, NJ: Prentice-Hall.

APPENDIX 6.A   A Craniofacial Screening Instrument*

Craniofacial Screening Profile   ☐ Examine

Name: _____ Sex: ☐ M ☐ F DOB: _____

Address: _____ Phone: _____

Parents: _____

Clinician: _____ Date: _____

Head Size: ☐ Normal	☐ Suspect Examples: Macrocephalus Microcephalus	**Hard Palate:** ☐ Normal ☐ Suspect Examples: Cleft or Hard Palate High Vaulted Hard Palate Notch in Posterior Palate
Facial Symmetry: ☐ Normal	☐ Suspect Examples: Hemifacial Microsomia	**Soft Palate:** ☐ Normal ☐ Suspect Examples: Cleft of Soft Palate Bifid Uvula Wide, Flat Uvula Fissured Uvula
Hair: ☐ Normal	☐ Suspect Examples: Sparse Coarse	**Faucial Pillars:** ☐ Normal ☐ Suspect Examples: Asymmetry of Pillars Webbed Pillars
Ears: ☐ Normal	☐ Suspect Examples: Microtia Skin Tags	**Lower Jaw:** ☐ Normal ☐ Suspect Examples: Micrognathia Prognathism
Eyes: ☐ Normal	☐ Suspect Examples: Hypertelorism Proptosis Coloboma	**Neck:** ☐ Normal ☐ Suspect Examples: Short Neck Webbed Neck
Nose: ☐ Normal	☐ Suspect Examples: Cleft Lip Nose Deviated Nasal Septum	**Shoulders:** ☐ Normal ☐ Suspect Examples: Raised Shoulder Blade
Lips: ☐ Normal	☐ Suspect Examples: Cleft Lip Notch in Upper Lip Lip Pits on Lower Lip	**Hands:** ☐ Normal ☐ Suspect Examples: Syndactyly Polydactyly
Alveolus and Teeth: ☐ Normal	☐ Suspect Examples: Cleft Alveolus Notch in Alveolus Hypodontia Hypoplasia of Maxilla	**Speech:** ☐ Normal ☐ Suspect Examples: Hypernasality NasalEscape Compensatory Articulation Nasal Turbulence Nasal Grimacing

1. Has the child undergone previous medical diagnosis or treatment for any type of suspected orofacial-craniofacial or related anomaly?
☐ No
☐ Yes—Description:
☐ Don't know

2. Is the child receiving special educational services at school?
☐ No
☐ Yes—Description:
☐ Don't know

3. Does the child require speech-language therapy at school?
☐ No
☐ Yes—Description:
☐ Don't know

4. Comments:

*Reproduced with permission from the American Cleft Palate-Craniofacial Association. Originally published in Coston, G. N., Sayetta, R. B., Friedman, H. I., Weinrich, M. C., Macera, C. A., Meeks, K., McAndrews, S. K., & Morales, K. S. (1992). Craniofacial screening profile: Quick screening for congenital malformations. *Cleft Palate-Craniofacial Journal, 29,* 87–91.

APPENDIX 6.B A Summary of Cranial Nerve Function for the Oral Musculature*

Cranial nerve	Muscles innervated	Movements and sensation innervated	Test procedure	Signs of lower motor neuron damage	Signs of upper motor neuron damage
V. Trigeminal	Masseter, tensor tympani, tensor veli palatine, mylohyoid, digastric (anterior belly)	Jaw closing, lateral jaw movement	Palpation of masseter; closing and lateralization against resistance	Weakness, jaw deviation to lesion side, atrophy	Mild, transitory weakness
VII. Facial	Orbicularis oculi and oris, zygomatic, buccinator, platysma, stylohyoid, stapedius, portion or digastric (posterior belly)	Forehead wrinkling, closing eyes, closing mouth, smiling, tensing cheeks, pulling down corner of mouth, tensing anterior neck muscles, moving stapedius to dampen ossicles; taste from anterior two-thirds of tongue and hard and soft palates	Observation of facial symmetry at rest; have patient wrinkle forehead, close eyes tightly, smile, pucker, and pull down lip corners; identification of tastes	Involvement of entire side of face, weakness, limited range of movement, decreased taste sensation	Complete involvement of lips and neck muscles, less involvement of eye-area muscles, little difficulty with forehead muscles; weakness; limited range of movement of affected muscles; decreased taste sensation
IX. Glossopharyngeal	Stylopharyngeus, otic ganglion, parotid salivary gland, part of the middle pharyngeal constrictor	Elevation of pharynx and larynx, pharyngeal dilation, and salivation; taste from posterior one-third of tongue; sensation from posterior tongue and upper pharynx	Tested with cranial nerve X for motor; sensory test for pharyngeal gag	—	—
X. Vagus	Inferior, middle, and superior pharyngeal constrictors; salpingopharyngeus, glossopalatine, pharyngopalatine, levator veli palatine, uvular, cricothyroid, thyroarytenoid, posterior and lateral cricoarytenoid, interarytenoid, and transverse and oblique interarytenoid muscles; various muscles of the viscera, esophagus, and trachea	Palatal elevation and depression, laryngeal movement, pharyngeal constriction, cricopharyngeal function	Observation of palatal movement, palatal gag reflex; laryngoscopic evaluation of vocal musculature; ability to change pitch; phonation time; assessment of swallowing	Absence of gag reflex, poor movement of palate or pharyngeal wall, absent or delayed swallow response, aspiration, breathy hoarse voice (may be improved by pushing effort)	Poor palatal or pharyngeal wall movement, harshness or strained-strangled voice quality, delayed or absent swallow reflex, aspiration

Cranial nerve	Muscles innervated	Movements and sensation innervated	Test procedure	Signs of lower motor neuron damage	Signs of upper motor neuron damage
XII. Hypoglossal	Superior longitudinal, inferior longitudinal, transverse, vertical, genioglossus, hyoglossus, and styloglossus	All tongue movements as well as some elevation of the hyoid bone	Observation for atrophy or fasciculations, as well as symmetry on protrusion; assessment for lateralization, protrusion, elevation, retraction (to observe range of movement); assessment of movement against resistance for strength testing on lateral, protrusion, and elevation movement; articulation testing	Atrophy, fasciculations, weakness, reduced range of movement, deviation of tongue to side of lesion, decreased tone, consonant imprecision	Weakness, reduced range of movement, deviation of tongue to contralateral side, increased tone, consonant imprecision

*Reproduced with permission from Love, R.J., & Webb, W.g. (1996). *Neurology for the speech-language pathologist* (3rd ed.) (p. 163–165). Boston: Butterworth–Heinemann.

APPENDIX 6.C   An Oral and Speech Motor Control Protocol*

Lips (CN VII)
Structure at rest

1. Symmetry
2. Relationship (open vs. closed)

Oral function

3. Rounding
4. Protrusion (blowing)
5. Retraction
6. Alternate pucker/smile
7. Bite lower lip
8. Lip seal
9. Puff cheeks
10. Open-close lips

Speech function

11. Rounding /oʊː/
12. Protrusion /uː/
13. Retraction /iː/
14. Alternate /u/, /i/
15. Bite lower lip /f/
16. Open-close lips /mʌ/

Mandible (CN V)
Structure at rest

17. Symmetry
18. Occlusion
19. Size (re: facial features)

Oral function

20. Excursion (click teeth 5×)

Maxilla
Structure at rest

21. Symmetry
22. Size

Teeth

23. Decay
24. Alignment
25. Gaps
26. Missing
27. Occlusion (re: maxillary teeth)

Tongue
Structure at rest

28. Symmetry
29. Carriage

30. Fasciculations
31. Furrowing
32. Atrophy
33. Hypertrophy

Oral function

34. Protrusion
35. Elevation to alveolar ridge
36. Anterior-posterior sweep
37. Interdental

Speech functions

38. Elevation to alveolar ridge: /n/, /t/, or /l/
39. Touch lateral edges of tongue to teeth: /s/ or /ʃ/
40. Interdental: /ɵ/
41. Posterior tongue to palate: /k/ or /g/

Velopharynx
Structure at rest

42. Symmetry
43. Uvula
44. Tonsils
45. Vault height
46. Palatal juncture (palpate)

Oral function

47. Blow on cold mirror
48. Suck through a straw

Speech functions

49. /aː/
50. /ha.ha.ha/

Larynx-Respiration (CN X)
Structure at rest

51. Posture during quiet breathing

Oral function

52. Cough, laugh, or cry

Speech function

81. Maximum phonation time (in seconds): /aː/
53. Pitch variation
54. Loudness variation
55. /ha.ha.ha/

Coordinated speech movements

56. (82)[a] /pʌ/ repetitions
57. (83)[a] /tʌ/ repetitions
58. (84)[a] /kʌ/ repetitions

59. (85)[a] /pɔrɔkɔk/ repetitions
60. (86)[a] patticake repetitions
61. You
62. Top
63. Beef
64. Fume
65. Cowboy
66. Band-aid
67. Half-time
68. Banana
69. Kitty cat
70. Puppy dog
71. Communicate
72. 1950
73. Potato head
74. Winnie the Pooh

Speech sample
Prosody

75. Rate
76. Intonation

Voice

77. Pitch
78. Loudness
79. Quality
80. Nasal resonance

[a]*Items 56–60 are scored for articulatory accuracy, and items 82–86 for mean number of repetitions per second over 3 seconds.*

*Reproduced with permission from Robbins, J., & Klee, T. (1987). Clinical assessment of oropharyngeal motor development in young children. *Journal of Speech and Hearing Disorders, 52*, 271–277.

APPENDIX 6.D Orofacial Examination Checklist*

Orofacial Examination Checklist

Client name:_____ Age:_____

Date:_____

Examiner:_____

I. Facial characteristics
  A. General appearance; normal color _____; normal symmetry _____; adenoid facies _____; other _____
  _____

  B. Frontal view
    1. Eye spacing: normal (one eye apart) _____; hypertelorism _____; other _____
    2. Zygomatic bones: normal _____; hypoplasia _____; other _____
    3. Nasal area: septum (straight) _____; or deviated _____; nares _____; columella _____; septum/turbinate relationship _____; turbinate color _____; other notations _____
    4. Vertical facial dimensions:
      a. Upper (40% of face) _____; other notations _____
      b. Lower (60% of face) _____; other notations _____
    5. Lips: Cupid's bow present _____; muscular union _____; neuromotor functioning—/i/ _____; /u/ _____; /p-p-p/ _____; other notations_____
    _____

  C. Profile
    1. Normal (straight or convex) linear relationship between bridge of nose, to base of nose, to chin _____
      maxilla _____; maxilla _____
      retrusion protrusion
      mandible _____; mandible _____
    2. Mandibular plane: normal _____; steep _____; flat _____

  D. General notations:_____
II. Intraoral characteristics
  A. Dentition
    1. General hygiene: good _____; needs improvement _____; caries _____; gingival hyperplasia or recession_____
    2. Occlusal relationships ("bite on your back teeth" and separate cheek from teeth with tongue depressor)
      a. First molar contacts:
        Class I—normal molar occlusion (mandibular molar is one-half tooth ahead of maxillary molar)
        _____

Class I malocclusion (normal molar relationship with variations in other areas of dentition) _____

_____

Class II malocclusion (maxillary ahead of mandibular first molar) _____

Class III malocclusion (mandibular molar more than one-half tooth ahead of maxillary molar)

_____

b. Biting surfaces: normal vertical overlap (overbite)_____;
   excessive vertical overlap A _____/ P _____;
   normal horizontal overlap (overjet) _____; excessive
   horizontal overlap A _____/ P _____; crossbite
   (mandibular tooth or teeth outside or wider than maxillary counterpart, or maxillary tooth or teeth inside mandibular counterpart) _____; notation of teeth involved
   _____; open bite (gap between biting surfaces) A
   _____/ P _____

c. Sibilant production with teeth in occlusion: normal /s/
   _____; /z/ _____

B. Hard palate ("extend your head backward")
   1. Midline coloration: normal (pink and white) _____; abnormal (blue tint) _____
   2. Lateral coloration: normal _____; torus palatinus (blue tint surrounding a raised midline bony growth) _____
   3. Posterior border and nasal spine: normal _____; short
      _____
   4. General bony framework: normal _____; submucous cleft
      _____; cleft _____; repaired cleft _____; other
      _____
   5. Palatal vault: normal relationship between maxillary arch/flat
      vault _____; narrow maxillary arch/high vault _____;
      wide maxillary arch/flat vault _____; other_____
   6. General notations: _____

      _____

C. Soft palate or velum (Examiner's eye level should be at client's mouth level. Client's head erect, mouth three-fourths open, and tongue not extended out of mouth.)
   1. Midline muscle union (say "ah"): normal (whitish-pink tissue line) _____; submucous cleft (blue tint with A-type configuration during phonation) _____; cleft _____;
      repaired cleft _____
   2. Length: effective (closure of nasopharyngeal port possible during phonation) _____; ineffective (hypernasality noted) _____
   3. Velar dimple (where elevated soft palate buckles during phonation): normal 80% of total velar length (or 3–5 mm above tip of uvula) _____; other notations _____

      _____

   4. Velar elevation: normal (up to plane of hard palate) _____;
      reduced _____; other _____

      _____

    5. Range of velar excursion (up and back stretching during pho-nation): excellent _____; moderate _____; minimal _____

    6. Presence of hypernasality during counting: 60s _____; 70s _____; 80s _____; 90s _____

    7. General notations: regarding air loss on unphonated sounds (nasal emission) and nasal resonance on phonated sounds _____

D. Uvula
    1. Shape: normal _____; bifid _____; other _____
    2. Position: midline _____; lateral _____

E. Fauces
    1. Open isthmus _____; tonsillar obstruction of isthmus _____

    2. Tonsil coloration: normal (pinkish) _____; inflamed _____

F. Pharynx
    1. Depth between velar dimple and pharyngeal wall on "ah": normal _____; deep _____; other _____
    2. Passavant's pad: present during physiologic activity? _____
    3. Adenoidal surgery (ask client): intact _____; removed _____; date of tonsil/adenoid removal _____;
    4. Gag response: positive _____; negative _____; weak _____
    5. General notations: _____
_____

G. Tongue
    1. size: normal _____; macroglossia (rare) _____; micro-glossia _____
    2. Diadochokinetic rate—an estimate of neuromotor maturation for speech (observe consistency and pattern of rapid move-ments during the 15-repetition sequence)
        a. Normal movement patterns: tuh _____; luh _____; kuh _____; puh-tuh-kuh _____; describe varia-tions _____
        b. Mandibular assist: normal (until age 7 $\frac{1}{2}$) _____; possi-ble neuromotor delay for speech (after age 7 $\frac{1}{2}$) _____
    3. Lingual frenum: normal (tongue tip to alveolar ridge when mouth is one-half open) _____; short _____
    4. General notations: _____
_____

III. General observations and other findings

Orofacial Examinations Checklist: Short Form

I. Facial characteristics
  A. Frontal view: eye spacing; zygomatic bones; nasal area; vertical dimensions; lips
  B. Profile: straight/convex; excessively convex; concave

II. Intraoral characteristics
  A. Dentition—general
    1. Occlusal relationships—anterior and posterior

2. Bite—normal: excessive overbite or overjet; open bite; cross-bite
3. Sibilant production/teeth relationships: /s/; /z/; /f/; /v/
B. Hard palate—bony shelf formation
   1. Coloration—midline; lateral
   2. Bony midline (palpate): normal; submucous cleft (short)
   3. Contour—vault/maxillary arch relationship
C. Soft palate or velum
   1. Midline muscle union—complete; submucous cleft
   2. Length at rest and effective length during phonation
   3. Location of dimpling on velum from nasal spine to uvula tip
   4. Velar elevation and range of velar excursion
   5. Acoustic correlates: amount of nasality during counting in 60s, 70s, 80s, and 90s
D. Uvula—shape and position
E. Fauces—isthmus opening and coloration; tonsils intact?
F. Pharynx
   1. Depth between velar dimple and pharyngeal wall on "ah"
   2. Observation of Passavant's pad during function
   3. Ask client if adenoids removed and subsequent speech status
   4. Gag response
G. Tongue
   1. Size related to oral environment
   2. Diadochokinetic rate on tuh; luh; kuh; puh-tuh-kuh
   3. Lingual frenum
III. General observations and other findings

---

*Reproduced with permission from Mason, R.M., & Simon, C. (1977). An oro-facial examination checklist. *Language, Speech, and Hearing Services in the Schools, 8,* 155–163.

APPENDIX 6.E Normative Syllable Repetition Rates (Diadochokinesis) for Children and Adults*

	Syllable patterns								
Age (years)	pʌ	tʌ	kʌ	fʌ	lʌ	pʌt	pʌkə	tʌkə	pʌtəkə
6.0	4.2	4.1	3.6	3.6	3.8	2.0	1.9	1.9	1.0
7.0	4.7	4.1	3.8	3.7	3.8	2.0	1.9	1.9	1.0
8.0	4.8	4.6	4.2	4.1	4.4	2.4	2.1	2.1	1.2
9.0	5.0	4.9	4.4	4.4	4.4	2.5	2.3	2.3	1.3
10.0	5.4	5.3	4.6	4.8	4.8	2.7	2.3	2.3	1.4
11.0	5.6	5.6	5.0	5.0	5.3	3.1	2.6	2.6	1.5
12.0	5.9	5.7	5.1	5.4	5.4	3.2	2.6	2.7	1.6
14.0	6.1	6.1	5.4	5.6	5.7	3.6	2.9	2.9	1.8
Adults	6.0–7.0[a]	6.0–7.0[a]	5.5–6.5[a]	6.4[b]	6.5[b]	4.6[c]	—	—	2.5

[a]Approximate range of means from Figures 3, 4, and 5.
[b]From Sigurd (1973).
[c]From Tiffany (1960).

*Reproduced with permission from Kent, R. D., Kent, J. F., & Rosenbeck, J. C. (1987). Maximum performance tests of speech production. *Journal of Speech and Hearing Disorders, 52,* 367–387.

Index

Page numbers followed by *t* indicate tables.

Fine motor skills, development of, 8
Fisher-Logemann Test of Articulation, 43
Fistula, palatal, 199
Fluency, evaluation of, 163, 164–174, 181–182, 210–211. *See also* Stuttering, assessment of; *specific tests*
Frenchay Dysarthria Assessment, 209

Genioglossus muscle, 191
Glossopalatine muscle, 191
Glossoptosis, 192
Goldman-Fristoe Test of Articulation, 37, 39
Graphophonemic analysis, 90
Gross motor skills, development of, 8

Hard palate, mechanism of, 198–200
Hoarseness, 22
Hyoglossus muscle, 191

ICIDH-2. *See* International Classification of Functioning and Disability (ICIDH-2)
Impairment, defined, 77–78
Independent analysis, 34
Indirect study methods, of physiological testing, 19
Inhalation/exhalation cycle, 205–206. *See also* Breathing
Inspiration, muscles of, 205. *See also* Breathing
Internal intercostals, 205–206
International Classification of Functioning and Disability (ICIDH-2), 77
Interpersonal skills, and diagnosis, 10
Interpretation, in diagnosis, 23–24
Interviews, in assessment of language, 82, 99–100

Jitter, as acoustic measure, 22

Language
    assessment of, 77–95, 101–104, 113f, 115, 117. *See also* Child speech disorder
    contextual measurements in, 89–91
    cultural considerations and, 79–80
    decontextualized measurement and, 91–94
    framework for, 80, 81f
    observation and, 80–87, 95t
    observation of participation and, 87–89
Language samples, in assessment of language functions, 82–84, 101–104

Laryngopharynx, 203
Lingual frenum, differential diagnosis of, 192
Lingual tonsil, 204
Lips, mechanism of, 188–190
Lobulation, 192
Loudness, assessment of, 175

Macroglossia, 192
Magnetic resonance imaging (MRI), in diagnosis, 21
Malocclusion, 194, 196–197
Medical records, and case history, 7
Microdontia, 198t. *See also* Teeth, mechanism of
Microglossia, 192
Minnesota Test for Differential Diagnosis of Aphasia (MTDDA), 123–127
Motor speech disorders, 189
    assessment of, 208–209, 210, 211
MRI. *See* Magnetic resonance imaging (MRI), in diagnosis
MTDDA. *See* Minnesota Test for Differential Diagnosis of Aphasia (MTDDA)
Multiple-branching. *See* Arborization

Naming, 127, 131, 142, 143, 144, 147, 152
    pictures, 124, 139–141
Narrative analysis, and dynamic assessment of language functions, 85t
Nasopharynx, 203
Natural Process Analysis, 34
Normative sample, in tests, 14

Observation
    and assessment of child speech disorders, 107–111
    and assessment of language functions, 80–87, 87–89, 95t
Oligodontia, 198t. *See also* Teeth, mechanism of
OMD. *See* Oral myofunctional disorders (OMD)
Open bite, 196
Oral and Speech Motor Control Protocol, 225–227
Oral examination
    commercial tests used in, 208–213. *See also specific tests*
    cranial nerves and, 188, 191–192, 199, 201, 204, 206, 223–224
    of breathing, 204–207
    of hard palate, 198–200
    of lips, 188–190
    of pharynx, 203–204